T0358644

Posterior Capsular Rupture

A Practical Guide to Prevention and Management

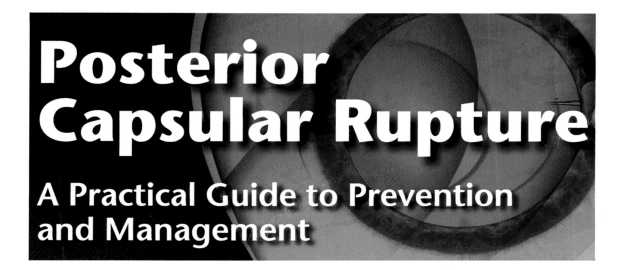

Posterior Capsular Rupture

A Practical Guide to Prevention and Management

EDITOR

AMAR AGARWAL, MS, FRCS, FRCOphth

Chairman and Managing Director
Dr. Agarwal's Group of Eye Hospitals
and Eye Research Centre
Chennai, India

ASSOCIATE EDITOR

SOOSAN JACOB, MS, FRCS, DNB, MNAMS

Senior Consultant Ophthalmologist
Dr. Agarwal's Group of Eye Hospitals
and Eye Research Centre
Chennai, India

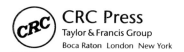

CRC Press
Taylor & Francis Group
Boca Raton London New York

CRC Press is an imprint of the
Taylor & Francis Group, an **informa** business

First published 2014 by SLACK Incorporated

Published 2024 by CRC Press
2385 NW Executive Center Drive, Suite 320, Boca Raton FL 33431

and by CRC Press
4 Park Square, Milton Park, Abingdon, Oxon, OX14 4RN

CRC Press is an imprint of Taylor & Francis Group, LLC

Library of Congress Cataloging-in-Publication Data

Posterior capsular rupture : a practical guide to prevention and management / [edited by] Amar Agarwal.
    p. ; cm.
  Includes bibliographical references and index.
  ISBN 978-1-61711-071-9 (alk. paper)
  I. Agarwal, Amar.
  [DNLM: 1. Cataract Extraction--methods. 2. Posterior Capsular Rupture, Ocular--therapy. 3. Intraoperative Complications. 4. Phacoemulsification--methods. 5. Posterior Eye Segment--surgery. WW 260]
  RE451
  617.7'42059--dc23
                    2013016028

ISBN: 9781617110719 (pbk)
ISBN: 9781003525813 (ebk)

DOI: 10.1201/9781003525813

Additional resources can be found at
https://www.routledge.com/9781617110719

DEDICATION

This book is dedicated to Gábor B. Scharioth, MD, PhD, from Germany, for being such a great friend and coming all the way to India to teach me how to perform canaloplasty and the proper usage of the glaucolight, and for showing the world that intrascleral haptic fixation is the way to go.

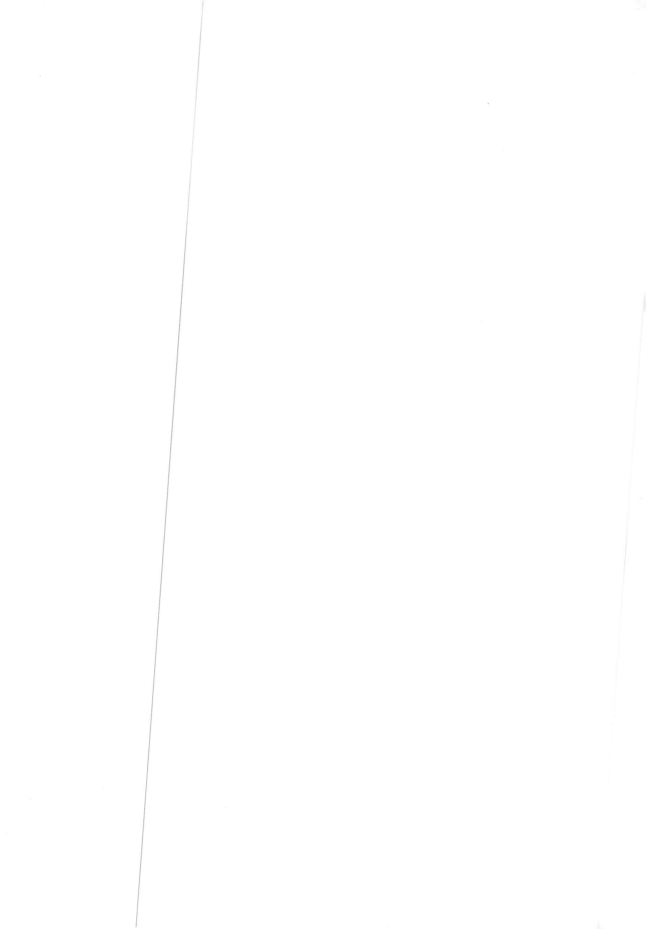

Contents

Acknowledgment

Nothing in this world moves without HIM, thus this book was written only through HIM.

ABOUT THE EDITORS

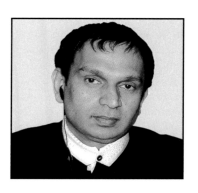

Amar Agarwal, MS, FRCS, FRCOphth is the Chairman and Managing Director of Dr. Agarwal's Group of Eye Hospitals and Eye Research Centre in India, which includes 55 eye hospitals; President of the International Society of Refractive Surgery (ISRS); and Secretary General of the Indian Intraocular Implant and Refractive Society (IIRSI).

Dr. Agarwal is the pioneer of phakonit, which is phaco-emulsification with needle incision technology. This technique became popularly known as bimanual phaco, microincision cataract surgery (MICS), or microphaco. He is the first to remove cataracts through a 0.7-mm tip with the technique called *microphakonit*. He also discovered no-anesthesia cataract surgery and FAVIT, a new technique to remove dropped nuclei. The air pump, which was a simple idea of using an aquarium fish pump to increase the fluid into the eye in bimanual phaco and coaxial phaco, has helped prevent surge. This built the basis of various techniques of forced infusion for small-incision cataract surgery. He also discovered a new refractive error called *aberropia*. He was also the first to perform a combined surgery of microphakonit (700-micron cataract surgery) with a 25-gauge vitrectomy in the same patient, thus creating the smallest incisions possible for cataract and vitrectomy. He was also the first surgeon to implant a new mirror telescopic intraocular lens for patients suffering from age-related macular degeneration (AMD). He also was the first in the world to implant a glued intraocular lens (IOL), whereby a posterior chamber IOL is fixed in an eye without the capsule using fibrin glue. The Malyugin ring (MicroSurgical Technology, Redmond, WA) for small-pupil cataract surgery was also modified by him as the Agarwal modification of the Malyugin ring for miotic pupil cataract surgery with posterior capsular defects. Dr. Agarwal's Eye Hospital has also, for the first time, performed an anterior segment transplantation in a 4-month-old child with anterior staphyloma. The turnaround technique for intrastromal ring segments being managed if passed through a false channel creation as well as the glued endocapsular ring for subluxated cataracts has also been started in Dr. Agarwal's Eye Hospital. Dr. Agarwal pioneered the technique of IOL scaffold in which retained nuclear fragments are emulsified by using a 3-piece IOL as a scaffold in an eye with posterior capsular rupture to prevent the nucleus fragments from dropping into the vitreous. He has combined glued IOL and IOL scaffold in cases of posterior capsular rupture where there is no iris or capsular support in a new technique termed the *glued IOL scaffold*.

Dr. Agarwal has received many awards for his work in ophthalmology, most significantly, the Casebeer Award, Barraquer Award, and the Kelman Award. His videos have won many awards at the film festivals of the American Society of Cataract and Refractive Surgery (ASCRS), the American Academy of Ophthalmology (AAO), and the European Society of Cataract & Refractive Surgeons (ESCRS). He has written more than 55 books which have been published in English, Spanish, and Polish. Dr. Agarwal also trains doctors from all over the world in the Eye Research Centre on phaco, bimanual phaco, LASIK, and retina. He is a Professor of Ophthalmology at Ramachandra Medical College in Chennai, India. The Web site for Dr. Agarwal's Eye Hospital is www.dragarwal.com.

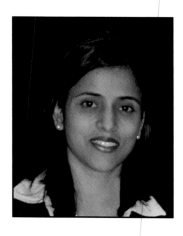

Soosan Jacob, MS, FRCS, DNB, MNAMS is a Senior Consultant Ophthalmologist in Dr. Agarwal's Eye Hospital, Chennai, India. She is a gold medalist in ophthalmology. She has won many international awards for video films and challenging cases at prestigious international conferences such as American Society of Cataract and Refractive Surgery (ASCRS), American Academy of Ophthalmology (AAO), World Ophthalmology Congress (WOC), and the European Society of Cataract and Refractive Surgeons (ESCRS). Dr. Jacon was awarded the prestigious John Henahan award for Young Ophthalmologist given by *EuroTimes* at the ESCRS Annual Meeting in 2011 and is one of the only 2 two-time winners of the prestigious Golden Apple award for the Challenging Cases Symposium in Cataract Surgery at the ASCRS. Dr. Jacob was also awarded the Special Gold Medal of the Indian Intraocular Implant and Refractive Society (IIRSI). Her videos have been featured videos and selected as Editor's Choice on the AAO, International Society of Refractive Surgery, Eyetube, and Ocular Surgery News (OSN) Web sites. She is a noted speaker and has conducted courses and delivered lectures in numerous national and international conferences. She has special interest in cutting edge surgical techniques for cataract, cornea, glaucoma, and refractive surgery including intra-stromal ring segments, collagen cross linking, subluxated cataracts, and new refractive solutions.

Dr. Jacob was the first to bring out the concept of anterior segment transplantation, a procedure in which the cornea, sclera, an artifical iris, pupil, and IOL are transplanted *en bloc* in patients with anterior staphyloma. She also devised a new surgical technique for ptosis in which the sling surgery can be done with a 1-stab incision rather than 3, thus improving the postoperative cosmetic appearance of the patient. She has devised 2 new techniques— the turnaround technique and the double pass turnaround technique for successful completion of femtosecond laser-assisted Intacs implantation in eyes with false channel dissection for both symmetric and asymmetric Intacs segments. She has also described new techniques of relaxing Descemetotomy for tractional Descemet's detachment and YAG/needle Descemetopuncture for bullous Descemet's detachment and has proposed a new classification system and treatment algorithm for Descemet's membrane detachments. She has developed an innovative technique for sutureless fibrin glue-assisted transscleral fixation of the capsular bag and its contents using a glued endocapsular ring, which makes safe phacoemulsification in subluxated cataracts possible and provides good intraoperative and postoperative safety and stability. Dr. Jacob won the ASCRS award for this procedure. She has also described a new contact lens-assisted crosslinking (CACXL) technique for use in keratoconic eyes with thin corneas where conventional crosslinking is not possible. In addition, Dr. Jacob described a single stab trabeculectomy technique for easy and rapid trabeculectomy surgery associated with less scarring and no subconjunctival dissection.

Dr. Jacob has written numerous articles and chapters in textbooks published by international and national publishers and she has been listed as the editor for 11 textbooks in ophthalmology. She has written numerous invited articles published in the Ophthalmology press. Her column, "Eye on Technology" is published in EuroTimes, the monthly magazine of the European Society of Cataract and Refractive Surgery. She is amongst the senior faculty for the Diplomate of National Board postgraduate training program and the phacoemulsification and LASIK training program for doctors outside of India. She is an Editorial Board member of the *Ocular Surgery News, Asia-Pacific Edition,* and an executive committee member of the Indian Intra-ocular Implant and Refractive Society. Her life and work has been featured on the cover page of *Ocular Surgery News* in the article, "Ophthalmic Innovator balances love of surgery, research and teaching" and in the prestigious *Cataract and Refractive Surgery Today* "5Q" interview.

CONTRIBUTING AUTHORS

Ashvin Agarwal, MS *(Chapter 13)*
Dr. Agarwal's Group of Eye Hospitals and Eye
    Research Centre
Chennai, India

Athiya Agarwal, MD, DO *(Chapter 8)*
Dr. Agarwal's Group of Eye Hospitals and Eye
    Research Centre
Chennai, India

Balamurali Krishna Ambati, MD, PhD
    (Chapter 12)
Moran Eye Center
University of Utah
Salt Lake City, Utah

J. Fernando Arevalo, MD, FACS *(Chapter 17)*
Executive Vice President of the Pan-American
    Association of Ophthalmology
Arlington, Texas
Chief of Vitreoretinal Division, Senior
    Academic Consultant
The King Khaled Eye Specialist Hospital
Riyadh, Kingdom of Saudi Arabia
Professor of Ophthalmology
Wilmer Eye Institute
The Johns Hopkins University
Baltimore, Maryland

Fernando A. Arevalo, BS *(Chapter 17)*
Retina and Vitreous Service
Clínica Oftalmológica Centro Caracas
Caracas, Venezuela

Clement K. Chan, MD, FACS *(Chapters 15 and
    18)*
Medical Director
Southern California Desert and Inland Retina
    Consultants
Palm Desert, California
Associate Clinical Professor
Department of Ophthalmology
Loma Linda University
Loma Linda, California

Garry P. Condon, MD *(Chapter 15)*
Allegheny Ophthalmic & Orbital Associates
Pittsburgh, Pennsylvania

Yassine Daoud, MD *(Chapter 11)*
Wilmer Eye Institute
The Johns Hopkins University
Baltimore, Maryland

Carlos F. Fernandez, MD *(Chapter 17)*
Retina and Vitreous Service
Clinica Oftalmologica Oftalmolaser
Lima, Peru

William J. Fishkind, MD, FACS *(Chapter 1)*
Co-Director
Fishkind, Bakewell, Maltzman
Eye Care and Surgery Center
Tucson, Arizona
Clinical Professor of Ophthalmology
The University of Utah
Salt Lake City, Utah
Clinical Professor of Ophthalmology
The University of Arizona
Tucson, Arizona

Sadeer B. Hannush, MD *(Foreword)*
Attending Surgeon
Wills Eye Institute
Department of Ophthalmology
Jefferson Medical College
Medical Director
Lions Eye Bank of Delaware Valley
Philadelphia, Pennsylvania

Thomas Kohnen, MD, PhD, FEBO *(Chapter 9)*
Professor and Chair
Department of Ophthalmology
Goethe University
Frankfurt, Germany

Dhivya Ashok Kumar, MD *(Chapter 2)*
Dr. Agarwal's Group of Eye Hospitals and Eye
    Research Centre
Chennai, India

Michael Lawless, MBBS, FRANZCO, FRACS
  (Chapter 14)
Medical Director
Vision Eye Institute
Sydney, Australia

Boris Malyugin, MD, PhD (Chapter 3)
Professor of Ophthalmology
S. Fyodorov Eye Microsurgery Complex State
  Institution
Moscow, Russian Federation

Kevin M. Miller, MD (Chapter 5)
Kolokotrones Professor of Clinical
  Ophthalmology
Jules Stein Eye Institute
David Geffen School of Medicine at the
  University of California, Los Angeles
Los Angeles, California

Zoltán Z. Nagy, MD, PhD, FEBO, DSc
  (Chapter 14)
Professor of Ophthalmology
Semmelweis University
Budapest, Hungary

Thomas A. Oetting, MS, MD (Chapter 10)
University of Iowa
Iowa City, Iowa

Marko Ostovic, MD (Chapter 9)
Department of Ophthalmology
Goethe University
Frankfurt, Germany

Som Prasad, MS, FRCSEd, FACS, FRCOphth
  (Chapter 7)
Consultant Ophthalmologist
Eye Department
Arrowe Park Hospital
Wirral, United Kingdom

Bryce R. Radmall, MD (Chapter 12)
Intermountain Medical Center
Murray, Utah

Shetal M. Raj, MS (Chapter 4)
Iladevi Cataract and IOL Research Centre
Raghudeep Eye Clinic
Memnagar, Ahmedabad, India

Brian C. Stagg, MD (Chapter 12)
Moran Eye Center
University of Utah
Salt Lake City, Utah

Walter J. Stark, MD (Chapter 11)
Wilmer Eye Institute
The Johns Hopkins University
Baltimore, Maryland

Abhay R. Vasavada, MS, FRCS
  (Chapters 4 and 6)
Iladevi Cataract and IOL Research Centre
Raghudeep Eye Clinic
Memnagar, Ahmedabad, India

Vaishali A. Vasavada, MS (Chapter 6)
Iladevi Cataract and IOL Research Centre
Raghudeep Eye Clinic
Memnagar, Ahmedabad, India

PREFACE

Regardless of the number of years in practice or the number of cases performed, the prevention and management of surgical complications remains the primary challenge for any surgeon. Although directly impacted by surgical technique, patient selection, and underlying disease processes, some complications inevitably arise even in the perfect candidate undergoing the procedure.

Although posterior capsular rupture management has evolved rapidly over the past 3 decades, so has the technical complexity of the interventions performed. As such, the surgeon must be ever cognizant of the potential complications associated with these evolving techniques. In this book on posterior capsular rupture, we have produced a sentinel collection of practical clinical strategies to which the surgeon can adhere and from which the surgeon can benefit. In doing so, not only will risks and complication rates be reduced, but they will also improve surgeons' diagnostic and therapeutic outcomes.

We wish that this book remain a fundamental reference for the management of posterior capsular rupture and hope that along with the interactive Web site, it will serve you, dear reader, as an excellent resource and guide for enhancing your practice.

Amar Agarwal, MS, FRCS, FRCOphth
Soosan Jacob, MS, FRCS, DNB, MNAMS
Dr. Agarwal's Group of Eye
Hospitals and Eye Research Centre
Chennai, India

FOREWORD

The Merriam-Webster dictionary defines "pioneer" as a person or group that originates or helps open up a new line of thought or activity or a new method or technical development. The same dictionary defines "Renaissance man" as a person who has wide interests and is an expert in several areas. Professor Amar Agarwal is indeed both a pioneer and Renaissance man. Over the past 2 decades Dr. Agarwal has investigated, developed, perfected, and taught many new ophthalmic surgical techniques from ultra small incision phacoemulsification (microphakonit) to Intralase assisted endothelial keratoplasty and, what he will likely be identified with for years to come, the fibrin sealant scleral fixated posterior chamber intraocular lens implant, more commonly known as the "glued IOL." He has freely shared his knowledge with the international ophthalmic community in scores of courses, live surgeries, peer reviewed publications, textbooks, and personal communications. To date, Dr. Agarwal has authored 55 books and trained close to 700 ophthalmologists from 6 continents who have visited him at his eye hospital in Chennai, India. Not to be outdone by the great ophthalmic innovators of the past half century, Dr. Agarwal and colleagues at his namesake eye hospital have many inventions and discoveries to their names including, but not limited to, the 5-mm optic rollable IOL, the concept of aberropia as a refractive error, and the glued IOL. This has not been overlooked by the international ophthalmic community. Dr. Agarwal has received many awards including the Barraquer, Casebeer, and Kelman awards. Perhaps the greatest honor of all is Dr. Agarwal's election as President of the International Society of Refractive Surgery (ISRS).

One of every cataract surgeon's daunting tasks and challenges is the anticipation, avoidance, and management of the ruptured posterior capsule. Again, Dr. Amar Agarwal comes to the rescue of his colleagues worldwide. In this book, Dr. Agarwal uses his encyclopedic knowledge to delineate a thoughtful approach to this surgical problem. In the first section, the guest authors describe the anticipation and prevention of posterior capsule rupture including the approach to posterior polar cataracts, the small pupil, intraoperative floppy iris syndrome (IFIS), and subluxated cataracts. This is followed by a section on the management of the rupture, vitrectomy techniques, and salvaging lens material. The third section goes over implantation of posterior chamber lenses in the setting of limited or no posterior capsular support, including Dr. Agarwal's own glued IOL technique. In the fourth and final section, Dr. Agarwal and his guest authors describe the complications associated with cases of posterior capsule rupture including dislocated IOLs, corneal damage, chronic inflammation and cystoid macular edema, and the dreaded postoperative endophthalmitis. Management algorithms are carefully delineated.

This latest addition to Dr. Agarwal's textbook publications is a must-read for any serious cataract or anterior segment eye surgeon who wishes to gain command of one of the most vexing surgical challenges in our subspecialty and to offer solutions in the interest of giving our patients the best chance for recovery of good vision. The book will undoubtedly become a major reference for trainees and practicing ophthalmologists alike. It is the latest contribution to the ophthalmic community worldwide from Dr. Agarwal, the pioneer and Renaissance man.

Sadeer B. Hannush, MD
Attending Surgeon, Wills Eye Institute
Department of Ophthalmology, Jefferson Medical College
Medical Director, Lions Eye Bank of Delaware Valley
Philadelphia, Pennsylvania

I

Prevention of Posterior Capsular Rupture

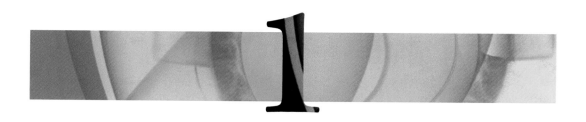

Understanding the Phacoemulsification Machine

Instrumentation and Techniques to Prevent and Manage Rupture of the Posterior Capsule

William J. Fishkind, MD, FACS

Modern phaco machine technology upgraded the phaco handpiece to the role of our most diverse and elegant handheld instrument. It can be used to both prevent tears in the capsule during phaco and it can be reprogrammed to minimize further damage if the capsule should rupture.

OVERVIEW

The patient will have the best visual result when the phaco energy delivered to the anterior segment is minimized. In addition, phaco energy should be directed into the nucleus, which will avoid injury to iris blood vessels, trabecular meshwork, and the endothelium. Finally, skillful emulsification will lead to shorter overall surgical time. Therefore, a lesser amount of irrigation fluid will pass through the anterior segment.

Normally, all phaco procedures have 2 phases. The first is the creation of fragments, which requires sculpting or chopping. The second phase is the removal of the fragments in a controlled approach. Occlusion is mandatory to move fragments to the iris plane. Fragment removal is assisted by partial occlusion phaco.

All phaco techniques are preceded by capsulorrhexis, cortical cleaving hydrodissection, and removal of the anterior cortex and epinucleus to expose the endonucleus.

Agarwal A.
Posterior Capsular Rupture: A Practical Guide to Prevention and Management (pp 3-17).
© 2014 Taylor & Francis Group.

DIVIDE-AND-CONQUER PHACO

Sculpting

To concentrate cavitational energy into the nucleus, a 0-, 15-, or 30-degree tip turned bevel down should to be utilized. Zero or low vacuum (depending on the manufacturer's recommendation) is mandatory for bevel-down phaco to prevent occlusion. Occlusion, at best, will cause excessive movement of the nucleus during sculpting. At worst, occlusion occurring near the equator or deep within the nucleus may capture nucleus, adherent cortex, capsule, and vitreous. This can be an origin of tears in the equatorial or posterior bag early in the phaco procedure.

After the groove is judged to be adequately deep (approximately 3-phaco tip diameters deep), the bevel of the tip should be rotated to the bevel-up position and vacuum will be increased. This will improve visibility and prevent the risk of phaco through the posterior nucleus and posterior capsule. Sculpting is assisted by the use of panel-control continuous phaco because the nucleus is held in place by the capsular bag. Therefore, pressure against the nucleus will allow a jackhammer effect to occur to emulsify a groove.

If micropulse phaco is used for sculpting, duty cycles with longer power "on" than power "off" should be selected. This will allow phaco to proceed with clean emulsification and avoid pushing the nucleus ahead of the phaco tip, potentially damaging the zonules. When the initial groove is judged adequate, the nucleus is rotated 90 degrees and another groove is created. Next, a 180-degree rotation allows access for creation of the final groove.

Quadrant and Fragment Removal

The grooves are expanded by cracking a fragment, which is then mobilized to the level of the iris. The tip selected, as noted previously, is retained. Vacuum and flow are increased to reasonable limits governed by the machine being used. The limiting factor to these levels is the development of surge. Therefore, the use of micropulse phaco or nonlongitudinal phaco is best used at this stage. The bevel of the tip is turned toward the quadrant or fragment. Low pulse or burst power is applied at a level high enough to emulsify the fragment without driving it away from the phaco tip.

Epinucleus and Cortex Removal

If cortical cleaving hydrodissection has been performed, the endonucleus is removed first, as noted previously. The result is a shell of epinucleus and cortex. For removal of the epinucleus and cortex, the vacuum is decreased while flow is maintained. This will allow for grasping of the epinucleus just deep enough to the anterior capsule to avoid contact with it. The low vacuum will help to hold the epinucleus on the phaco tip without breaking off chunks. High vacuum results in pieces of the epinucleus and cortex breaking off, making it more difficult to remove. With the fluid parameters balanced, the epinucleus/cortex scrolls around the equator and can be pulled to the level of the iris. There, low power pulsed or hyperpulse phaco is used for emulsification.

STOP AND CHOP PHACO

Groove creation is performed as noted. Once a single deep groove is adequate, vacuum and flow are increased to improve the holding capability of the phaco tip. The nucleus is rotated 90 degrees and the phaco tip is driven into the mass of 1 heminucleus using pulsed linear phaco. The sleeve should be 1 mm from the base of the bevel of the phaco tip to create adequate exposed needle length for sufficient holding power. Excessive phaco energy application is to be avoided, as this will cause the nucleus immediately adjacent to the tip to be emulsified. Thus, the gap created in the vicinity of the tip is responsible for interfering with the seal around the tip, as well as the capability of the vacuum to hold the nucleus. The nucleus will then pop off the phaco tip, making chopping more difficult. With a good seal, the heminucleus can be drawn toward the incision, and the chopper can be inserted at the endonucleus–epinucleus junction. The chopper is then drawn down and to the left while the phaco tip is pushed up and to the right. This will result in chopping of the heminucleus.

After the first chop, a second similar chop is performed so the heminucleus is divided into 3 pieces. One of the pie-shaped pieces of nucleus thus created is elevated to the iris plane (occlusion is utilized to move fragments) and removed with low-power hyperpulsed phaco or nonlongitudinal phaco, as discussed in the "Divide-and-Conquer Phaco" section. Each fragment and the remaining heminucleus are removed in turn. Epinucleus and cortex removal are also performed as noted previously.

Phaco Chop

Phaco chop requires no sculpting. Therefore, the procedure is initiated with high vacuum and flow and linear pulsed or micropulse phaco power. Nonlongitudinal phaco does not work well for the actual chopping, as the shaving movement of the phaco tip prevents an adequate vacuum seal to assist chopping and fragment mobilization. For a 0-degree tip, especially when emulsifying a hard nucleus, a small trough may be required to create adequate room for the phaco tip to push deep into the nucleus. For a 15- or a 30-degree tip, the tip should be rotated bevel down to engage the nucleus. The phaco tip should be encased within the endonucleus with the minimal amount of power necessary. All chopping procedures require 1 mm of exposed phaco tip to create adequate holding power for chopping. If the phaco tip is inserted into the nucleus with excess power, the adjacent nucleus will be emulsified, creating a poor seal between the nucleus and tip. This will make it impossible to remove fragments, as the tip will just "let go" of the nuclear material. In addition, the bevel should be turned toward the fragment to create a seal between the tip and fragment, allowing vacuum to build and create holding power.

Horizontal Chop

A few bursts or pulses of phaco energy will allow the tip to be encased within the nucleus. It then can be drawn toward the incision to allow the chopper access to the epi/endo nuclear junction. The chopping instrument is passed over the nucleus and under the anterior capsule into this junction. It may be helpful to rotate the chopper to the horizontal position as it passes below the anterior capsule. If the nucleus comes off the phaco tip, excessive power has produced a space around the tip, thus impeding vacuum holding power as noted previously. Pulling the chopper down and to the left and pushing the phaco tip up and to the right will generate the first chop. Minimal rotation of the nucleus will allow for the creation of the second chop. The first pie-shaped piece of nucleus is mobilized with high vacuum and elevated to the iris plane. There it is emulsified with low-linear hyperpulse or nonlongitudinal power, high vacuum, and moderate flow.

Vertical Chop

Once the phaco tip is embedded within the nucleus as previously described, a sharp Nichamin chopper (Katena Products, Denville, NJ) is pushed down into the mass of the nucleus at the same time the phaco tip is elevated. The chopper is then drawn down and to the left and the phaco tip

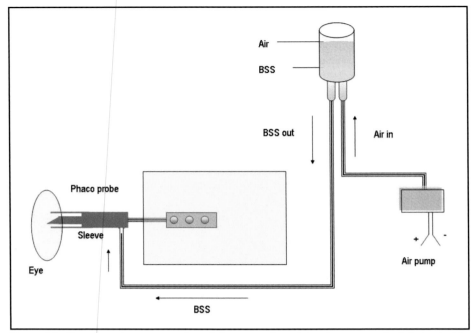

Figure 1-1. Diagrammatic representation of the connection of the air pump to the infusion bottle. (Reprinted with permission from Agarwal A, Lindstrom R. *Microincisional Cataract Surgery: The Art and Science.* Thorofare, NJ: SLACK Incorporated; 2010:24.)

up and to the right. This creates a cleavage plane in the nucleus. With a second chop, the fragment created is mobilized to the iris plane and removed as noted previously. When the nucleus is noted to be hard, the process of rotation and vertical chopping is repeated until the entire nucleus is chopped. Usually at this point the nucleus loses its rigidity, allowing the segments to be mobilized without difficulty.

MICROINCISIONAL PHACO

The development of micropulse and nonlongitudinal phaco ("cold phaco") has led to the performance of phaco through increasingly small incisions with tighter irrigation sleeves, no irrigation sleeves, and decreased inflow.

Bimanual Microincisional Phaco

Two incisions are created 90 degrees apart. The incision size is dependent on the instrumentation used. It is best to use 22-gauge (0.7 mm) instruments requiring sub 1-mm incisions. This is the smallest incision yet for performing cataract surgery and the surgical procedure is referred to as *microphakonit,* or sub 1-mm cataract surgery. This was first performed by Dr. Amar Agarwal.[1] There is no irrigating sleeve on the phaco tip. One needs to have gas-forced infusion, as shown by the air pump (Figure 1-1), which was developed by Dr. Sunita Agarwal for biaxial phaco.[2] The instrumentation for this procedure is important, and the relationship between the instrument and incision size is essential. If the wound is too tight, it is difficult to manipulate the instruments. If the wound is too large, excessive outflow permits chamber shallowing with an unstable anterior segment. The instruments can be moved forward and backward through the incisions without creating corneal distortion. If the instruments are angled in the incision, sufficient corneal distortion occurs and the procedure is appreciably more difficult to perform. The irrigating chopper should be parallel to the iris and above it. The inflow current thus created tends to wash fragments toward the unsleeved phaco tip. The small incisions cause less disruption of the blood aqueous barrier and are more stable and secure. In current practice, a new incision is created for intraocular lens (IOL) implantation. In the future, with insertion of an IOL through the sub 1-mm incision, there should be less disruption of ocular integrity, less risk of postoperative wound complications, and immediate return to full activities for the patient.

Microincisional Coaxial Phaco

A thin-walled, flared, 21-gauge phaco tip and thinner irrigation sleeve is available for Infinity Vision System machines (Alcon Laboratories, Fort Worth, TX), which now permits phaco though a 2.2-mm incision. Despite the smaller incision, inflow is adequate to maintain a deep anterior chamber. The procedure is no more difficult than when performed through a 2.8-mm incision. Alcon Laboratories also manufactures a single-piece acrylic IOL and injector, which is capable of implanting the IOL through the 2.2-mm unenlarged incision.

Similar to phaco, anterior chamber stability during irrigation/aspiration (I/A) is due to an equilibrium of inflow and outflow. Wound outflow can be minimized by using a soft sleeve around the I/A tip. Combined with a small incision (2.8 to 3 mm), a deep and stable anterior chamber will result. Linear vacuum allows the cortex to be grasped under the anterior capsule with low vacuum and drawn into the center of the pupil at the iris plane. There, in the safety of a deep anterior chamber, vacuum can be increased and the cortex aspirated.

Bimanual I/A is also a viable procedure. A 21-gauge irrigating cannula provides inflow through one paracentesis while an unsleeved 21-gauge aspiration cannula is used through the opposite paracentesis. The instruments can be easily switched, making removal of stubborn cortex considerably easier.[3]

MACHINE SETTINGS

Table 1-1 makes obvious the complexity of the machine settings for the Ellips FX (Abbott Medical Optics, Santa Ana, CA). Every machine, by virtue of its pump dynamics, software, tubing, foot pedal, venting, and tuning will have distinctive settings. The optimum approach to define the settings that would be most advantageous to the surgeon is to work with the manufacturer's surgical representative to fine-tune settings.

CAPSULAR TEARS

The capsule can tear at any time during phaco surgery. If the capsule tears before phaco is initiated, the following lists the likely origins:

- Extension of an anterior capsulorrhexis tear centripetally around the equator into the posterior capsule.

- Hydrodissection, with or without capsular block, "blowing out" the anterior capsule or posterior capsule.

- Pre-existing posterior capsule pathology, such as a posterior polar cataract or a vitrectomy, where the posterior capsule sustained damage from the vitrector.

If the capsule tears during the phaco procedure, the likely origins are as follows:

- Aspirating the capsule either posteriorly or at the equator and energizing phaco energy resulting in an immediate tear at the site of occlusion; the likelihood of rupture of the vitreous face is high.

TABLE 1-1. MACHINE SETTINGS FOR ELLIPS FX

ELLIPS FX	ASPIRATION RATE	VACUUM	POWER	NOTES
Hard Chop				
Unoccluded	32 cc/min panel Ramp 35%	340 mm Hg panel	50% linear	Whitestar (WS) 90-cm bottle height Kick 6 to 12 (0% to 80%)
Occluded Threshold 200	28 cc/min 30% ramp speed	340 mm Hg linear	50% linear 6 long pulses per second	90-cm bottle height
Chop				
Unoccluded	32 cc/min panel Ramp 30%	325 mm Hg linear	40% linear WS On/Off = 8/4 PPS = 83 Duty cycle 67%	92-cm bottle height Kick 5 fixed 0% to 80%
Occluded Threshold 200	30 cc/min linear Ramp 30%		40% linear 6 long pulses per second	90-cm bottle height
Soft Chop				
Unoccluded	30 cc/min panel Ramp 40%	260 mm Hg linear	35% linear Variable WS On/Off = 10/12, 10/10, 10/6, 10/4 PPS = 45, 50, 62, 71 Duty cycle = 45, 50, 63, 71	90-cm bottle height Kick 6 to 12 (0% to 80%)
Occluded Threshold 200	28 cc/min panel	20% ramp speed 90-cm bottle height Occlusion threshold 175 mm Hg	35% linear 6 LPPS	

(continued)

TABLE 1-1 (CONTINUED). MACHINE SETTINGS FOR ELLIPS FX

ELLIPS FX	ASPIRATION RATE	VACUUM	POWER	NOTES
Epinucleus				
Unoccluded	30 cc/min panel	300 mm Hg linear	10% linear	90-cm bottle height Kick 6 to 12 (0% to 80%)
Occluded Threshold 150	22 cc/min panel	300 mm Hg linear	10% Linear 4 LPPS	
I/A 1 (Max Vac)	26 linear Ramp 75% Non-zero start 10 cc/min	600 linear Non-zero start 50 mm Hg		80-cm bottle height
I/A 2 (Cap Vac)	5 panel Ramp 25%	5 linear		50-cm bottle height
I/A 3 (Viscoelastic Removal)	38 panel Ramp 80%	500 linear Non-zero start 50 mm Hg		90-cm bottle height

ELLIPS FX	ASPIRATION RATE	VACUUM	CUTS PER MINUTE (CPM)	NOTES
Vitrectomy 1	20 panel	300 linear	1500 panel	Bottle 90 cm C-I/A (Cut-I/A)
Vitrectomy 2	20 panel	300 linear	1500 panel	Bottle 90 cm I/A-C (I/A-Cut)
Diathermy	50% linear			
Foot Pedal Settings	0% to 5% foot position zero	5% to 19% foot position 1	19% to 72% foot position 2	72% to 100% foot position 3

PPS = pulse per second
Max Vac = Maximum vacuum
C-I/A = Cut-irrigation/aspiration
I/A-C = Irrigation/aspiration-cut

- Attempting to phacoemulsify a mature cataract through a capsulorrhexis that is too small, causing a tear in the anterior capsule extending into the posterior capsule. The vitreous face may remain intact.
- Aspirating the posterior capsule during a surge; the likelihood of rupture of the vitreous face is high.

If the capsule tears during I/A, the likely origins are as follows:

- Aspirating the capsule instead of cortex, thereby pulling and tearing it.
- Aspirating the capsule instead of cortex and having a sharp burr in the aspiration orifice tear it.
- Aspirating cortex and continuing to aspirate the attached capsule until it tears.
- Aspirating ophthalmic viscosurgical device (OVD) and, secondary to surge, aspirating and tearing the posterior capsule.

Although there are many variations on the aforementioned themes, they represent a distillation of the problems and allow the surgeon to separate the scenarios required for successful outcome.

Some universal principles affect outcome in all cases of torn capsule. The following is a list of universal principles:

- Attempt to maintain a small wound and a closed chamber.
- Attempt to prevent enlargement of the tear.
- If the anterior capsule and capsulorrhexis are intact, attempt to preserve the integrity of the anterior capsule and capsulorrhexis to provide support for a sulcus-fixated and/or bag-fixated IOL.
- Attempt to avoid rupture of the vitreous face.
- Never withdraw the phaco tip in the presence of a torn capsule without first filling the anterior chamber with OVD. Without OVD, the forceful shallowing of the anterior chamber will likely produce extension of the tear, and, in all probability, will rupture the vitreous face.
- Prevent loss of the nucleus into the vitreous.
- Have unpreserved triamcinolone acetonide injectable suspension (Triesence), 40 mg/mL available.
- Have a vitrectomy kit containing the vitrector, tubing, irrigating cannulas, needle holder, and suture readily available and in 1 location.

MANAGEMENT OF A TEAR IN THE ANTERIOR CAPSULE WITHOUT A TEAR IN THE POSTERIOR CAPSULE

Once a tear of the anterior capsule is recognized (Figures 1-2A and 1-2B), it is imperative to maintain a stable anterior chamber. For example, pressure posteriorly (from the phaco tip pushing posteriorly while attempting to chop the nucleus) or pressure anteriorly (from removing the phaco tip and allowing the vitreous to move anteriorly) is adequate stimulus to tear the capsule through the equator and into the posterior capsule.

Therefore, the anticipated approach is to maintain a stable anterior chamber. Actual machine settings are dependant on the machine, grade of cataract, the surgical technique used, and the surgeon. However, certain generalizations hold true.

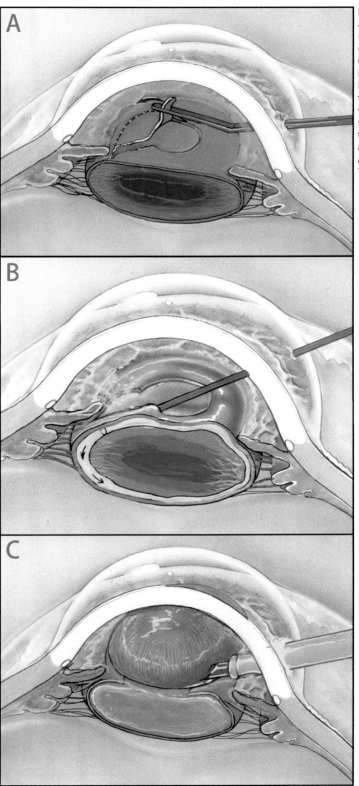

Figure 1-2. Equatorial tear in the anterior capsule during (A) capsulorrhexis, and (B) hydrodissection, and (C) Viscoat sandwich. The dispersive OVD is under the cataract, which has been prolapsed into the anterior chamber. OVD will now be placed above the nucleus to suspend it for removal without putting pressure on the capsular bag. (Reprinted with permission from Fishkind WJ, ed. *Complications in Phacoemulsification: Avoidance, Recognition, and Management.* New York, NY: Thieme Publishers; 2002.)

For a Hard or Moderate Cataract

Chop

Confirm there is 1 mm of exposed phaco tip. This is important to establish so that the surgeon can verify that there is sufficient holding power for chopping maneuvers. If there is not enough exposed tip, simply slide the sleeve back a little bit more. Switch to panel control and turn the power to 50% or more. Use longitudinal power (ie, not OZil or elliptical). Increase vacuum slightly (the author's preferred setting is 340 mm Hg), increase flow slightly (the author's preferred setting is 30 cc/min unoccluded, increasing to 38 cc/min with occlusion to improve holding ability), lower the irrigating bottle 20 cm (the author's preferred setting is 70 cm). These changes will cause the tip to energize at 50% power immediately on entering foot pedal position 3. The increased flow and vacuum allow the tip to pass into the central nucleus without posterior pressure. The decreased inflow also decreases posterior pressure. The avoidance of OZil or elliptical power affects the nonlongitudinal movement of the phaco tip. This brings about a tight fit between the tip and the nucleus for improved holding power, which is required for either vertical or horizontal chopping. With the tip firmly embedded in the nucleus and with the foot pedal in position 2 so that vacuum holds the nucleus firmly on the phaco tip, the phaco tip can slightly lift the nucleus and vertical chopping can be accomplished within the confines of the capsular bag without putting pressure on the posterior capsule. The nucleus is rotated, and this process is repeated until the entire nucleus is chopped into small pieces and nuclear rigidity is disrupted. Then, the phaco machine is set to linear power with micropulse and/or nonlongitudinal power, if available. The power is decreased to 30%, and vacuum and flow are set to appropriate levels to prevent surge. The bottle remains in its position. Each fragment of nucleus is then elevated to the central pupil at the plane of the anterior capsule where it is emulsified.

Prior to removing the phaco tip, OVD is utilized to fill the anterior chamber. This prevents positive posterior pressure from moving the vitreous anteriorly and consequently enlarging the tear. It also prevents the initial infusion surge from the I/A tip from pushing the posterior capsule and the vitreous posteriorly and enlarging the tear.

Assuming the posterior capsule has remained intact, the cortex is removed with I/A. The cortical removal begins opposite from the anterior capsular rent. As the location of the rent is approached, the cortex is engaged with low-linear aspiration. As aspiration increases, the cortex is pulled toward the rent in an attempt to prevent enlargement. Venturi pump technology makes the aspiration control more precise in this situation.

Alternatively, a dispersive OVD can be used to fill the capsular fornices and can then be aspirated, revealing the cortex below and allowing for cortex removal in a more expanded capsular bag environment.

After IOL insertion, remaining OVD is removed with moderate linear vacuum and a lowered irrigation bottle. A more gentle method for removing the OVD is to remove it in aliquots by aspirating a few tenths of a cc in a 3-cc syringe with a 25-gauge cannula and then replacing the volume with balanced salt solution (BSS). This procedure is repeated until most of the OVD is removed.

Alternatively, bimanual I/A provides a nicely controlled environment for both the cortical clean-up and removal of the OVD. The larger fluid fluxes seen with coaxial I/A are avoided with this technique.

Divide-and-Conquer

Confirm there is 1 mm of exposed phaco tip. This is important to establish so there is sufficient grove depth for grooving maneuvers. If there is not enough exposed tip, simply slide the sleeve back a little bit more. Switch to panel control and turn the power to 100%. Use nonlongitudinal continuous power (ie, OZil or elliptical, if available). Decrease vacuum significantly so there is no tendency for the phaco tip to grab and pull the nucleus during grooving. Keep flow at the usual setting. It is important to have adequate inflow to cool the phaco tip. Lower the irrigating bottle 20 cm. These changes will cause the tip to energize at 100% power immediately on entering foot pedal position 3. The immediate power prevents the phaco tip from pushing the nucleus ahead and posteriorally of it, potentially further tearing the torn anterior capsule. The nonlongitudinal power assists in cutting the groove. The decreased inflow from the lower infusion bottle diminishes posterior pressure. Create the grove with minimal posterior pressure, shaving and deepening the grove gradually, dependent on the consistency of the nucleus. When groove depth is judged to be sufficient, gently rotate the nucleus 180 degrees in the plane of the capsular bag and complete the groove. For stop and chop, rotate the nucleus 90 degrees and proceed as indicated previously for chopping with the new machine settings. If continuing to divide-and-conquer, rotate the nucleus 45 degrees and create another groove. After all 8 groves are complete, they can be separated with minimal force and distance. The pie-shaped fragments thus produced are then emulsified at the plane of the anterior capsule in the mid-pupil with the settings as noted for chopping techniques.

Viscoat Sandwich

Another alternative to the aforementioned scenarios is to create a "Viscoat sandwich." Because there is already a tear in the anterior capsule, it is a straightforward procedure to mobilize the entire cataract into the anterior chamber. This is accomplished by injecting a dispersive OVD behind the cataract while simultaneously elevating the cataract into the anterior chamber. More OVD is placed over the nucleus to suspend it in the anterior chamber and protect the endothelium. The nucleus is then emulsified in the anterior chamber, using whatever technique is preferred. Obviously, this prevents any posterior pressure on the capsule, thus minimizing the risk of tear extension (Figure 1-2C).

It is important to have the nucleus immediately adjacent to the phaco tip when power is energized. The high power, moderate vacuum, low flow, and low-infusion bottle settings assist in pulling the nucleus into the phaco tip while maintaining a stable anterior chamber. In machines where torsional or elliptical nonlongitudinal and micropulse power settings are available, they should be utilized.

CAPSULAR TEARS DURING PHACO

As soon as the capsule tears during phaco, the normal fluid dynamics of the anterior segment are disturbed. The open capsule allows inflow fluid to flow through the rent into the vitreous. As a result, the irrigation inflow from the phaco sleeve will tend to push fragments away from the tip. This dynamic is so enhanced that it is difficult for aspiration forces to overcome it. In addition, hydration of the vitreous and turbulence brings vitreous into the anterior chamber where it is easily aspirated by the large-bore phaco tip. This occludes the needle orifice, making aspiration of the nucleus even more difficult. It may appear that the nucleus will not come up to the phaco tip or even be pushed away from it (Figure 1-3).[4]

To prevent this, the infusion bottle must be lowered significantly (approximately 70 cm). The aspiration flow rate and vacuum should also be lowered. If possible, dispersive OVD can be used to push vitreous posteriorly and to provide a barrier between the vitreous and the phaco tip. It also serves to elevate nuclear material above the plane of the anterior capsule where it can be emulsified. The anterior chamber can even be filled with OVD, as described by Dr. David F. Chang in the Viscoat trap technique.[5]

If there is already too much vitreous in the anterior chamber for the use of OVD, limited vitrectomy may be necessary to remove vitreous which would otherwise prevent aspiration of the nucleus. Excessive vitrectomy should be avoided at this stage, as it may possibly allow nucleus, or pieces of the nucleus, to fall into the vitreous. OVD can be then used as a barrier as described previously. The phaco tip should be placed adjacent to the nuclear fragment before aspiration is engaged. The

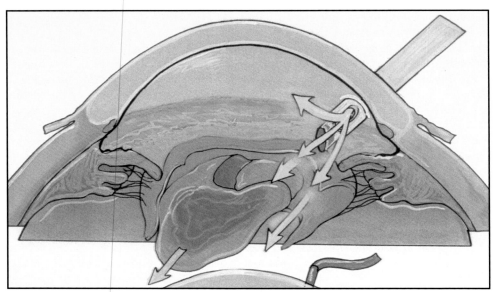

Figure 1-3. Once the posterior capsule is torn, its barrier effect is impaired. Inflow pushes lens material away from the phaco tip. (Reprinted with permission from Fishkind WJ, ed. *Complications in Phacoemulsification: Avoidance, Recognition, and Management.* New York, NY: Thieme Publishers; 2002.)

second instrument should be utilized to hold the fragment against the phaco tip, assuring it will be aspirated rather than vitreous. Only then can aspiration overcome inflow and allow emulsification of the remaining nucleus (Figure 1-4). If the nucleus begins to fall posteriorly, it must be secured with OVD and a Sheets' glide technique, as described by Michelson (Figure 1-5),[6] an Agarwal IOL scaffold technique, or a Kelman posterior assisted levitation (PAL) technique (Figure 1-6).[5]

Once the nucleus is removed, the cortex should be removed next. This can be done beautifully with a vitrector, which will allow for aspiration without cutting. For aspiration, set the foot pedal in position 2, and for cutting, set the foot pedal in position 3. The cortex can be aspirated without cutting and vitrectomy, with cutting, can be performed intermittently as necessary. Bimanual I/A would be the next best option for cortex removal. The absence of an irrigating sleeve and the separation of irrigation from aspiration prevent the irrigation fluid flow from pushing cortex away from the aspirating tip.

The last choice, obviously, is coaxial I/A. Again, it is advantageous to use a lowered infusion bottle, low aspiration flow rate (20 cc/min), and linear vacuum (300 to 500 mm Hg, maximum). The aspiration orifice should be placed close to the cortex to aspirate it preferentially over OVD and vitreous. Once cortex is engaged, the vacuum is progressively increased until aspiration is complete.

A thorough vitrectomy should be performed after all cortex is removed. Vitrectomy should also be performed intermittently whenever vitreous prevents either emulsification of nucleus or aspiration of cortex. In this case, the cutting mode of the vitrector should be engaged before the aspiration mode so as not to create vitreous traction. This is the C-I/A setting. Therefore, cutting is engaged in foot pedal position 2, and aspiration is engaged in foot pedal position 3. The cutting rate should be set as high as possible on older machines, usually 350 to 550 cuts per minute. On newer machines, cutting rates of 1500 cuts per minute actually allow sculpting of the vitreous and decrease the volume of vitreous removal. Vacuum of 100 to 125 mm Hg and aspiration flow of 20 cc/min are appropriate settings for vitrectomy. These parameters may be modified in different machines and with different pumps.

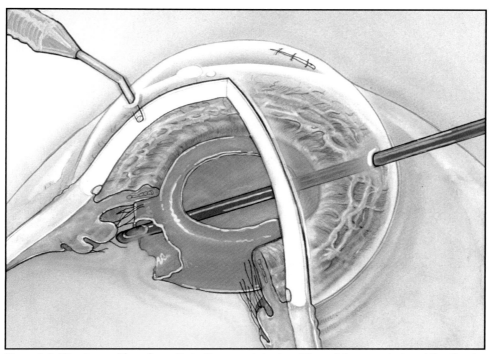

Figure 1-4. Vitrectomy with unsleeved irrigation cannula is placed through 1 paracentesis and the vitrector is placed through another paracentesis. The cutter passes through the tear in the capsule into the vitreous to minimize pulling the vitreous up into the anterior chamber. (Reprinted with permission from Fishkind WJ, ed. *Complications in Phacoemulsification: Avoidance, Recognition, and Management.* New York, NY: Thieme Publishers; 2002.)

Irrigation is provided by a 21-gauge cannula placed through the paracentesis. If a small paracentesis is initially created, it must be enlarged for cannula passage. Similarly, the vitrectomy instrument should be placed through a new paracentesis and appropriately sized. Alternatively, pars plana vitrectomy can be performed. Conversion to extracapsular cataract extraction is another alternative option.

Unpreserved triamcinolone acetonide injectable suspension 40 mg/mL is a superb adjunct to vitrectomy. It can be diluted 1 part to 4 parts BSS. Injected into the anterior chamber, it reveals residual vitreous and, importantly, vitreous strands incarcerated in the various incisions.

CONCLUSION

When challenged by a critical crisis such as the torn capsule, a carefully designed surgical plan is an enormous advantage. Understanding the principles of the fluid dynamics in the altered anterior segment may avert a major complication. Possessing the instruments to perform vitrectomy and being aware of the machine settings that will enhance the effectiveness of the instruments can salvage the visual outcome for the patient.

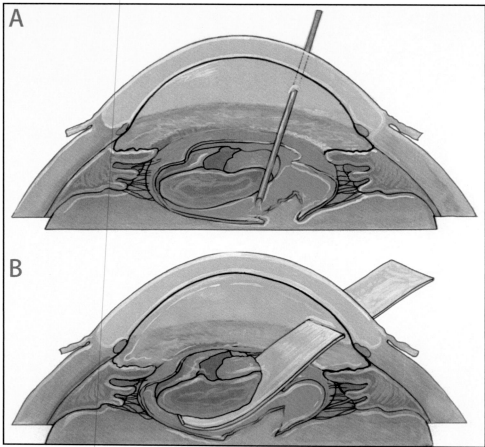

Figure 1-5. Michelson's Sheets' glide technique. The glide passes below the nucleus through the OVD to create a false posterior capsule, which allows the nucleus to be emulsified without dropping into the vitreous. (Reprinted with permission from Fishkind WJ, ed. *Complications in Phacoemulsification: Avoidance, Recognition, and Management*. New York, NY: Thieme Publishers; 2002.)

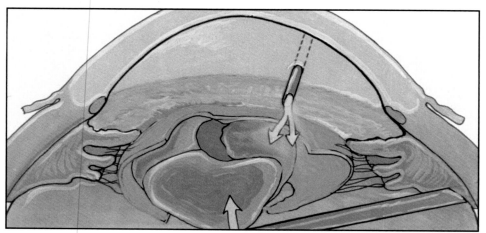

Figure 1-6. The Kelman PAL technique. A probe is placed through the pars plana and is used to lever the nucleus into the anterior chamber where it is trapped and secured. (Reprinted with permission from Fishkind WJ, ed. *Complications in Phacoemulsification: Avoidance, Recognition, and Management*. New York, NY: Thieme Publishers; 2002.)

REFERENCES

1. Agarwal A, Trivedi RH, Jacob S, et al. Microphakonit: 700 micron cataract surgery. *Clin Ophthalmol.* 2007;1(3):323-325.
2. Agarwal A, Agarwal S, Agarwal A, et al. Antichamber collapser. *J Cataract Refract Surg.* 2002;28(7):1085-1086.
3. Fishkind WJ. The phaco machine: understanding the equipment to take advantage of contemporary phaco techniques. In: Colvard MD, ed. *Achieving Excellence in Cataract Surgery.* D. Michael Colvard, MD, FACS. 2009;67-75.
4. Chang DF. Strategies for the difficult capsulorrhexis. In: Chang DF. *Phaco Chop: Mastering Techniques, Optimizing Technology, and Avoiding Complications.* Thorofare, NJ: SLACK Incorporated; 2004:143-162.
5. Chang DF. Strategies for managing posterior capsular rupture. In: Chang DF. *Phaco Chop: Mastering Techniques, Optimizing Technology, and Avoiding Complications.* Thorofare, NJ: SLACK Incorporated; 2004:212-217.
6. Michelson MA. Torn posterior capsule. In: Fishkind WJ, ed. *Complications in Phacoemulsification: Avoidance, Recognition and Management.* New York, NY: Thieme Publishers; 2002:127-129.

2

Posterior Capsular Rupture

Dhivya Ashok Kumar, MD and Amar Agarwal, MS, FRCS, FRCOphth

Any breach in the continuity of the posterior capsule is defined as a posterior capsular tear. Intrasurgical posterior capsule tears are the most common and can occur during any stage of cataract surgery.[1-3] The incidence of posterior capsule complications is related to the type of cataract and the condition of the eye. The incidence of complications increases with the difficulty of the case, and is further influenced by the level of experience of the surgeon. Timely recognition and planned management—depending on the stage of surgery during which the posterior capsule tear occurred—is required to ensure an optimal visual outcome.

COMMON RISK FACTORS FOR POSTERIOR CAPSULAR RUPTURE AND ENLARGEMENT

The following are common risk factors for posterior capsular rupture:
- Shallow anterior chamber
- Type of cataract or associated ocular condition
- Extended rhexis

Shallow Anterior Chamber

Intraoperative shallow anterior chamber could be due to a variety of reasons such as a tight lid speculum, tight drape, or pull from the collecting bag. In such instances, the precipitating factor can be easily removed. Variation in the amount of space in the anterior and posterior chambers may also result from changes in intraocular pressure (IOP) due to an alteration in the equilibrium between inflow and outflow of fluid. Diminished inflow may be secondary to insufficient bottle

Agarwal A.
*Posterior Capsular Rupture: A Practical Guide
to Prevention and Management* (pp 19-29).
© 2014 Taylor & Francis Group.

Figure 2-1. Hydrodelineation performed in a posterior polar cataract.

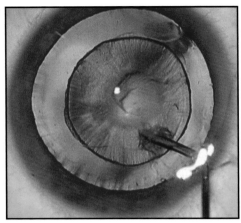

height, unnoticed empty bottle, tube occlusion or compression, excessively tight incision compressing the irrigating sleeve, or partial withdrawal of the phaco tip from the incision, causing the irrigating ports to come out of the incision. Excessive outflow may be caused by large incisions with leakage, high vacuum/flow parameters, or postocclusion surge. Use of gas-forced infusion or an air pump connected to the infusion bottle can usually avoid intraoperative shallowing of the anterior chamber.[1]

Type of Cataract or Associated Ocular Condition

A higher incidence of posterior capsular rupture and vitreous loss is seen in cataracts associated with pseudoexfoliation, diabetes mellitus, and trauma. Missing the diagnosis in a posterior polar cataract (Figure 2-1) can be catastrophic to the surgeon and the patient, as it is frequently associated with a weakened or deficient posterior capsule. Posterior lenticonus, cataract with persistent hyperplastic primary vitreous, cataract following vitreoretinal surgery, cataract in a high myopic patient, cataract in the presence of asteroid hyalosis, and mature and hypermature Morgagnian cataracts are some other types of cataracts associated with increased risk of posterior capsular rupture. Eyes with small pupils and other risk factors that make surgery more challenging can also increase the risk of posterior capsular rupture. The degree of surgeon experience is an important factor in preventing a posterior capsular rupture. Each of the aforementioned risk factors should be attended to in an appropriate manner. Avoid hydrodissection in patients with posterior polar cataract as it may cause hydraulic perforation at the weakened area of the capsule; only a carefully controlled hydrodelineation is preferred. One can also perform a gentle multiquadrant viscodissection under the anterior capsule in such a manner that the viscoelastic does not spread beyond the anterior rim of the capsule. This can prevent an accidental fluid wave from the phaco handpiece moving posteriorly and resulting in a posterior capsular rupture. If a capsular tear does occur, it is of prime importance not to withdraw the phaco handpiece suddenly but rather to maintain a closed system and prevent a sudden shallowing of the anterior chamber by injecting viscoelastic before withdrawing the phaco tip. This helps to tamponade the lens and vitreous backward when a capsular dehiscence is present.

Extended Rhexis

Extension of an anterior capsule tear can occur as a complication of standard phaco or micro-incision cataract surgery (MICS). This can occur during capsulorrhexis when an anterior capsular tear extends posteriorly to the posterior capsule. This situation can be managed by creating a nick

TABLE 2-1. SIGNS OF POSTERIOR CAPSULAR RUPTURE

1. Sudden deepening of the chamber with momentary expansion of the pupil.
2. Sudden, transitory appearance of a clear red reflex peripherally.
3. Apparent inability to rotate a previously mobile nucleus.
4. Excessive lateral mobility or displacement of the nucleus.
5. Excessive tipping of 1 pole of the nucleus.
6. Partial descent of the nucleus into the anterior vitreous space.
7. "Pupil snap sign"—sudden marked pupil constriction after hydrodissection.

on the anterior capsule using a cystotome, Vannas scissors (Appasamy Associates, Chennai, India), or vitreoretinal scissors and completing the capsulorrhexis from the opposite side. The viscoelastic in the anterior chamber is then expressed out to make the globe hypotonic. A gentle hydrodissection is performed at 90 degrees from the tear while pressing the posterior lip of the incision to prevent any rise in IOP. No attempt is made to press on the center of the nucleus to complete the fluid wave. The fluid is usually sufficient to prolapse one pole of the nucleus out of the capsular bag. If not, it is removed by embedding the phacoemulsification probe, making sure not to exert any downward pressure, and then gently pulling the nucleus anteriorly. No nuclear division techniques are tried in the bag. The entire nucleus is prolapsed into the anterior chamber and emulsified.

MANAGEMENT OF POSTERIOR CAPSULAR TEAR

Every surgeon should be aware of the signs of posterior capsular rupture (Table 2-1). Posterior capsular tears can occur during any stage of phacoemulsification surgery. However, tears occur most frequently during nuclear emulsification, as reported by Mulhern et al[4] (49%) and Osher and Cionni,[5] as well as during irrigation/aspiration (I/A), as reported by Gimbel.[6]

The following 3 possible situations can exist in a posterior capsular rent[7]:

1. Posterior capsular rupture with hyaloid face intact and nuclear material present.

2. Posterior capsular rupture with hyaloid face ruptured without luxation of nuclear material into the vitreous.

3. Posterior capsular rupture with hyaloid face ruptured and luxation of nuclear material into the vitreous.

Immediate precautions should be taken to not increase the size of the posterior capsular rupture or to further hydrate the vitreous. On noticing the posterior capsular rupture, the surgeon should immediately stop aspiration and resist the temptation to withdraw the phaco probe. Instead, dispersive ophthalmic viscosurgical device (OVD) is injected from the sideport to stabilize the anterior chamber and tamponade the vitreous, then the probe is removed, being careful to not be in foot pedal 2 position. Conventional management is to prevent the mixing of cortical matter with vitreous, prevent fragment drop, use dry aspiration where indicated, and perform bimanual anterior vitrectomy. In addition, if a posterior capsular rupture occurs during phacoemulsification, low flow parameters are advocated.

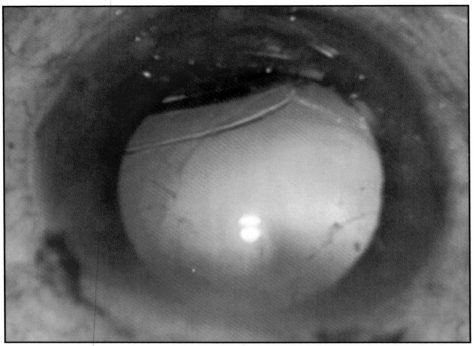

Figure 2-2. Posterior capsular rupture. Note the intraocular lens (IOL) sinking into the vitreous cavity. The white reflex indicates nuclear fragments dropped into the vitreous cavity. This patient was managed by vitrectomy, the fall-in vitreous (FAVIT) technique (removal of the nuclear fragments), and IOL repositioning into the sulcus.

REDUCE THE PARAMETERS

Lowering aspiration flow rate and decreasing the vacuum will control surge and allow the bottle to be lowered, thus diminishing turbulence inside the eye. If the nucleus is soft with only a small residual amount remaining and if the anterior hyaloid face is intact with no vitreous prolapse, dispersive OVD is used to tamponade the anterior vitreous face while the surgeon carefully continues the procedure. If vitreous is already present, special care must be taken to prevent hydration of the vitreous and additional vitreous prolapse into the anterior chamber or to the wound. A small amount of residual nucleus or cortex can be emulsified by gently bringing it out of the capsular bag and emulsifying it in the anterior chamber with dispersive viscoelastic coating the corneal endothelium. In the case of a small posterior capsular rupture and minimal residual nucleus (Figure 2-2), a dispersive viscoelastic is injected to plug the posterior capsular rupture. Subsequently, the nuclear material is moved into the anterior chamber with a spatula and emulsified. The recommended parameters are low bottle height (20 to 40 cm above the patient's head), low flow rate (10 to 15 cc/min), vacuum of approximately 100 to 200 mm Hg, and low ultrasound (20% to 40%).

Dry Cortical Aspiration

If there is only a small amount or no vitreous prolapse in the presence of a small capsular rent, a dry cortical aspiration with a 23-gauge cannula can be performed.

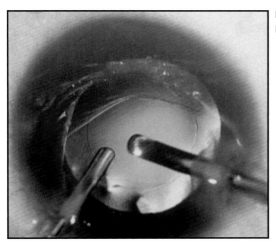

Figure 2-3. Bimanual vitrectomy is being performed in a posterior capsular tear with vitreous prolapse.

Viscoexpression

Viscoexpression is a method of removal of the residual nucleus by injecting viscoelastic underneath the nucleus as support, and the nucleus is expressed along with the viscoelastic.

Conversion to Extracapsular Cataract Extraction

If there is sizeable amount of residual nucleus, it is advisable to convert to a large-incision extracapsular cataract extraction (ECCE) to minimize the possibility of a dropped nucleus.

Anterior Bimanual Vitrectomy

Bimanual anterior vitrectomy is performed in eyes with vitreous prolapse (Figure 2-3). A 23-gauge irrigating cannula is used via a sideport incision. The irrigation bottle is positioned at the appropriate height to maintain the anterior chamber during vitrectomy. Vitrectomy should be performed with a cutting rate of 500 to 800 cuts per minute, an aspiration flow rate of 20 cc/min, and a vacuum of 150 to 200 mm Hg.

Anterior Chamber Cleared of Vitreous

Vitrectomy is continued in the anterior chamber and the pupillary plane. A rod swept through the anterior chamber can be used to check the presence of any vitreous strands; if present, the strands should be removed. Complete removal of the vitreous from the anterior chamber can be confirmed if you see a circular, mobile pupil and a complete air bubble in the anterior chamber. Preservative-free purified triamcinolone acetate suspension (Kenalog) is effective when used to identify vitreous strands, as described by Peyman et al (Figure 2-4).[8] Kenalog particles remain trapped on and within the vitreous gel, making them clearly visible.[9]

Suture the Wound

In cases of vitreous loss with posterior capsular rupture, it is recommended to suture the corneal wound as a prophylaxis to prevent infection. Remove any residual vitreous in the incision site in the main and sideports with a vitrector or remove it manually with Vannas scissors. As described previously, a blunt rod introduced via the sideport and swept to the center of the pupil over the surface of the iris can release these strands.

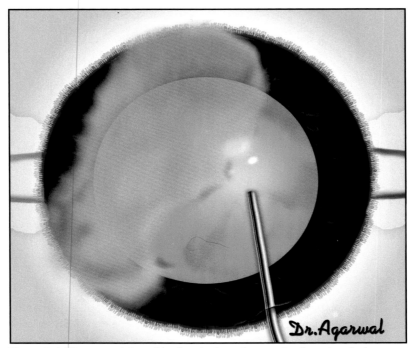

Figure 2-4. Vitreous staining with triamcinolone. Preservative-free triamcinolone acetonide suspension is injected intracamerally. The particles become enmeshed within the vitreous, making it difficult to visualize the vitreous strands. This helps with performing a thorough vitrectomy and completely removing all vitreous traction. All the granules should be removed at the end. (Reprinted with permission from Agarwal A. *Illustrative Guide to Cataract Surgery: A Step-by-Step Approach to Refining Surgical Skills*. Thorofare, NJ: SLACK Incorporated; 2012.)

TABLE 2-2. INTRAOCULAR LENS IMPLANTATION IN POSTERIOR CAPSULAR TEAR

1. Insertion and rotation of the IOL should always be away from the area of capsular tear.
2. The long axis of the IOL should cross the meridian of the posterior capsular tear.
3. In eyes with a posterior capsule tear (< 6 mm) with no vitreous loss, the IOL can be placed in the capsular bag.
4. In the presence of a posterior capsule tear (> 6 mm) with adequate anterior capsule rim, the IOL can be placed in the sulcus.
5. In deficient capsules, the glued IOL is a promising technique without the complications associated with sutured scleral fixated or anterior chamber IOLs.

INTRAOCULAR LENS IMPLANTATION

Depending on the state of the capsular bag and rhexis, the IOL is implanted in one of the manners described in the following paragraphs (Table 2-2).

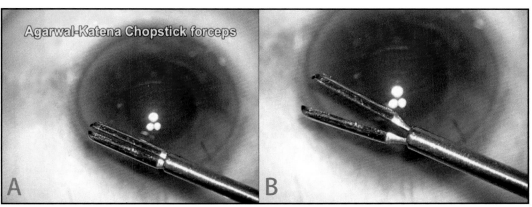

Figure 2-5. The Agarwal-Katena forceps. Reverse opening shown.

Eyes With Sufficient Capsular Support

In the Sulcus

If the rent is large and if sufficient capsular rim is available, the IOL can be placed in the sulcus. In cases with large posterior capsular rupture where conversion to ECCE was done, a rigid IOL can be placed in the sulcus over the residual anterior capsular rim with McPherson forceps (Appasamy Associates) holding the optic. The "chopstick technique" is another method of placing the IOL into the sulcus. The chopstick forceps (Agarwal-Katena forceps; Katena Products, Denville, NJ) (Figure 2-5) are used for IOL implantation with the chopstick technique. This technique refers to the IOL being held between the 2 jaws of the forceps. The advantage of using this technique is the smooth placement of the IOL into the sulcus without excess manipulation. Moreover, the IOL implantation is more controlled by using the forceps compared with other methods (Figure 2-6). A 3-piece foldable IOL can be placed in the sulcus when the incision has not been extended. A single-piece acrylic IOL should not be placed in the sulcus. In eyes with intraoperative miosis with posterior capsular rupture, the Agarwal-modified Malyugin ring can be used for pupillary dilatation. With this method,[10] a 6-0 polyglactic suture is placed in the leading scroll of the Malyugin ring and injected into the pupillary plane. The end of the suture stays at the main incision. Once in place, the ring produces a stable mydriasis of approximately 6 mm. The IOL can be implanted in the sulcus with good visualization, and this prevents inadvertent dropping of the iris expander into the vitreous during intraoperative manipulation.

In the Bag

In the presence of a small posterior capsular rupture with a mostly intact capsular bag, the IOL can be placed in the bag (Figure 2-7). An attempt can be made to convert the posterior capsular rupture into a primary posterior curvilinear capsulorrhexis. The foldable IOL can then be placed in the bag.

Eyes With Deficient Capsular Support

In eyes with insufficient anterior capsular support for sulcus placement of the IOL, there are different options for IOL placement. The authors' personal preference is the glued IOL technique of intrascleral haptic fixation.[11-13] Other options include sutured scleral fixated posterior chamber lenses, retroiridal fixation of posterior chamber IOLs, and anterior chamber IOLs.[14,15]

Figure 2-6. Chopstick technique. (A) The chopstick forceps are a reverse-acting, duck-billed forceps used to hold the IOL. The IOL is then inserted into the sulcus. The Y rod can be used to move the inferior iris out of the way to better see the anterior capsular flap. (B) The IOL is not released until it is completely placed within the sulcus. The broad jaws of the forceps hold the IOL firmly and prevents it from dropping down through the rent into the vitreous cavity. (Reprinted with permission from Agarwal A. *Illustrative Guide to Cataract Surgery: A Step-by-Step Approach to Refining Surgical Skills.* Thorofare, NJ: SLACK Incorporated; 2012.)

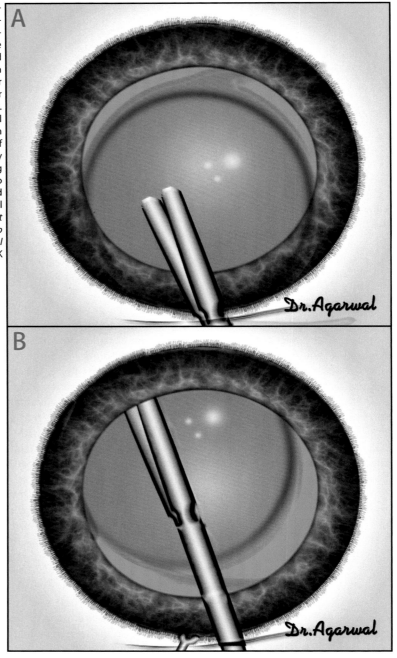

Sequelae After Posterior Capsular Rupture

Vitreous Traction

Incomplete vitrectomy can produce dynamic traction on the retina, leading to retinal breaks.

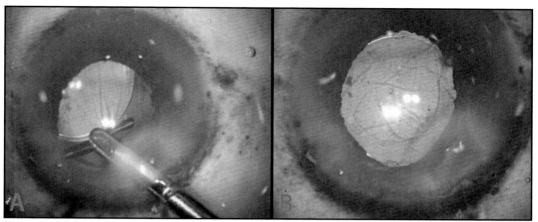

Figure 2-7. (A) A foldable IOL is placed into the sulcus with Agarwal-Katena forceps. (B) The IOL is well-centered on the capsular rim.

Retinal Detachment

Undetected, long-standing vitreous traction progresses to retinal break and detachment (Figure 2-8).

Macular Edema

Manipulation of the vitreous will increase not only the traction transmitted to the retina, but also the inflammation in the posterior segment and the risk of cystoid macular edema (CME).

Vitritis

Overenthusiastic use of viscoelastic in the vitreous can lead to sterile inflammation. Dropped residual cortex or nucleus can also present with postoperative vitritis.

Intraocular Lens-Related Complications

Improperly placed IOLs can lead to uveitis hyphema glaucoma (UGH) syndrome, lens-induced astigmatism and tilt, diplopia, subluxation of the IOL, and dislocation of the IOL into the vitreous cavity.

Conclusion

The occurrence of a posterior capsular rupture during cataract surgery is a serious complication. It is important for the surgeon to diagnose the occurrence of the posterior capsular rupture at an early stage to avoid further enlargement of the tear and associated vitreous complications. The primary goal at all stages is to remove the remaining nucleus, epinucleus, and cortex without causing vitreoretinal traction.

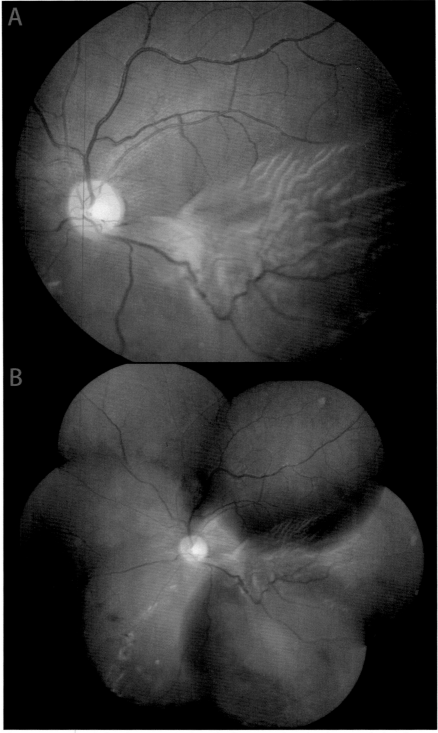

Figure 2-8. Retinal detachment. (A) Close fundus view showing the retinal detachment. (B) Montage showing the extent of the retinal detachment.

REFERENCES

1. Agarwal A. *Phaco Nightmares: Conquering Cataract Catastrophes*. Thorofare, NJ: SLACK Incorporated; 2006.
2. Agarwal S, Agarwal A, Agarwal A. *Phacoemulsification*. 3rd ed. New Delhi, India: Jaypee Brothers Medical Publishers; 2004.
3. Fishkind WJ. Facing down the 5 most common cataract complications. *Review of Ophthalmology*. 2001;8(10):37.
4. Mulhern M, Kelly G, Barry P. Effects of posterior capsular disruption on the outcome of phacoemulsification surgery. *Br J Ophthalmol*. 1995;79:1133-1137.
5. Osher RH, Cionni RJ. The torn posterior capsule: its intraoperative behaviour, surgical management and long term consequences. *J Cataract Refract Surg*. 1990;16:490-494.
6. Gimbel HV. Posterior capsular tears during phacoemulsification—causes, prevention and management. *Eur J Refract Surg*. 1990;2:63-69.
7. Vajpayee RB, Sharma N, Dada T, et al. Management of posterior capsule tears. *Surv Ophthal*. 2001;45:473-488.
8. Peyman GA, Cheema R, Conway MD, Fang T. Triamcinolone acetonide as an aid to visualization of the vitreous and the posterior hyaloid during pars plana vitrectomy. *Retina*. 2000;20:554.
9. Burk SE, Da Mata AP, Snyder ME, Schneider S, Osher RH, Cionni RJ. Visualizing vitreous using Kenalog suspension. *J Cataract Refract Surg*. 2003;29:645.
10. Agarwal A, Malyugin B, Kumar DA, Jacob S, Agarwal A, Laks L. Modified Malyugin ring iris expansion technique in small-pupil cataract surgery with posterior capsule defect. *J Cataract Refract Surg*. 2008;34(5):724-726.
11. Agarwal A, Kumar DA, Jacob S, et al. Fibrin glue–assisted sutureless posterior chamber intraocular lens implantation in eyes with deficient posterior capsules. *J Cataract Refract Surg*. 2008;34:1433-1438.
12. Agarwal A, Kumar DA, Prakash G, et al. Fibrin glue–assisted sutureless posterior chamber intraocular lens implantation in eyes with deficient posterior capsules [Reply to letter]. *J Cataract Refract Surg*. 2009;35:795-796.
13. Prakash G, Kumar DA, Jacob S, et al. Anterior segment optical coherence tomography–aided diagnosis and primary posterior chamber intraocular lens implantation with fibrin glue in traumatic phacocele with scleral perforation. *J Cataract Refract Surg*. 2009;35:782-784.
14. Bleckmann H, Kaczmarek U. Functional results of posterior chamber lens implantation with scleral fixation. *J Cataract Refract Surg*. 1994;20:321-326.
15. Numa A, Nakamura J, Takashima M, Kani K. Long-term corneal endothelial changes after intraocular lens implantation. Anterior vs posterior chamber lenses. *Jpn J Ophthalmol*. 1993;37:78-87.

Small Pupils and Intraoperative Floppy-Iris Syndrome

Boris Malyugin, MD, PhD

A clear and unobstructed view of the intraocular structures is a prerequisite for many surgical procedures.[1-6] Sufficient pupil dilation not only provides the surgeon access to the lens but also prevents posterior capsular rupture resulting from poor visualization and trauma to the delicate intraocular structures.

INTRAOPERATIVE FLOPPY-IRIS SYNDROME

Poor pupil dilation can be observed in cases complicated by pseudoexfoliation syndrome, uveitis, posterior synechiae, trauma, or previous intraocular surgery. Chang and Campbell[7] described intraoperative floppy-iris syndrome (IFIS) associated with systemic administration of the alpha-1A antagonists (tamsulosin hydrochloride and others). The intraoperative diagnostic triad of this symptom is fluttering and billowing of the iris stroma, significant tendency to iris prolapse through the main and/or sideport incisions, and progressive constriction of the pupil during surgery. The main cause of IFIS is thinning of the iris dilator muscle resulting in the changing of biomechanical properties and decreased rigidity of the iris tissue.

PHARMACOLOGICAL THERAPY

Pharmacological therapy with the use of nonsteroidal eye drops or strong mydriatics, such as phenylephrine 10%, is effective when administered preoperatively. Nevertheless, it cannot provide an adequate pupil aperture in all patients. Phenylephrine administration sometimes leads to unwanted ocular and systemic side effects.

Agarwal A.
Posterior Capsular Rupture: A Practical Guide to Prevention and Management (pp 31-39).
© 2014 Taylor & Francis Group.

SMALL PUPIL AND PHACOEMULSIFICATION

In small pupils the iris tissue is located closer to the phaco needle tip, which is the zone of the high-fluidic currents. That is why the iris has a high tendency to be aspirated into the ultrasound or irrigation/aspiration (I/A) handpiece. Decreasing flow parameters is an important factor in preventing iris damage during phacoemulsification. Central positioning and minimal movement of the handpiece are also important to prevent iris damage. Endocapsular lens nucleus fragmentation is much safer because the areas of the highest fluidic currents are located inside the capsular bag, away from the iris.

METHODS

The following methods may solve the problem of small pupils:
- Injection of intracameral mydriatic (nonpreserved epinephrine)
- Viscomydriasis (with high-viscosity ophthalmic viscosurgical device [OVD])
- Synechiolysis and/or pupillary membranectomy with spatula and forceps
- Mini sphincterotomies
- Pupillary stretching (if the pupil is very small)
- Use of mechanical pupil expansion devices such as iris hooks, pupil expansion rings, and the Malyugin ring

Mini Sphincterotomies

Mini sphincterotomies can be done with either Vannas scissors through the main incision or with vitreoretinal scissors placed through the paracentesis. Very small partial cuts, no larger than 0.75 mm in radial length, are made not extending beyond the sphincter tissue. As long as the incisions are kept very small, the pupil should be normal postoperatively—both functionally and esthetically. The disadvantage is that, to make the cuts throughout the whole circumference of the pupil, multiple additional corneal incisions for scissors introduction into the anterior chamber are necessary.

Mechanical Stretching of the Pupil

Mechanical stretching of the pupil is usually effective for small pupils with rigid iris tissue that is caused by prior miotic use, pseudoexfoliation, or posterior synechiae. Stretching can be achieved with the spatula, Sinskey hook (Katena Products, Denville, NJ), or special instrument (eg, Beehler pupil dilator [Moria, Doylestown, PA]) (Figure 3-1). Usually a pair of hooks, choppers, or similar instruments—introduced through 2 stab incisions in the cornea—engage the iris sphincter in the technique described by Miller and Keener.[8] The hooks are then pulled in opposite directions. This maneuver creates microscopic sphincter tears, which enlarge the pupil aperture. The main advantage of this procedure is that it is relatively simple and can be performed even without special instruments. Mechanical stretching of the pupil usually provides sufficient access to the lens and maintains the pupil diameter intraoperatively. The drawback of this technique is that it creates permanent damage to the iris sphincter. Microtears of the sphincter muscle are usually clinically asymptomatic, but they sometimes result in bleeding and pigment dispersion postoperatively.

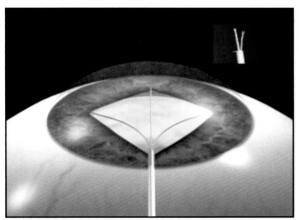

Figure 3-1. Tripronged pupil stretchers. (Reprinted with permission from Agarwal A. *Phaco Nightmares: Conquering Cataract Catastrophes.* Thorofare, NJ: SLACK Incorporated; 2006.)

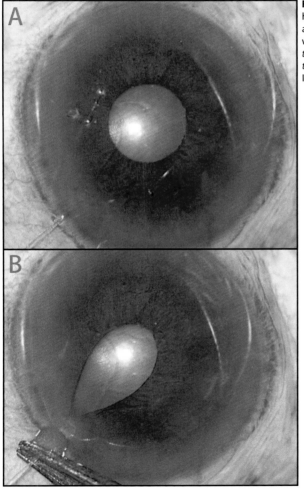

Figure 3-2. (A) A small pupil is seen. (B) An iris hook is inserted through the corneal paracentesis and the pupillary margin is engaged. (Reprinted with permission from Agarwal A. *Illustrative Guide to Cataract Surgery: A Step-by-Step Approach to Refining Surgical Skills.* Thorofare, NJ: SLACK Incorporated; 2012.)

Iris Hooks

Retracting the iris tissue, rather than cutting it, is simple and results in a better postoperative pupil appearance (Figure 3-2). Dr. Richard Mackool was the first to describe a 4-point iris retractor

Figure 3-2 (continued). (C) Consecutive iris hooks are inserted to obtain a square or diamond configuration. (D) Once adequate pupillary dilatation is obtained, phaco can be continued. (Reprinted with permission from Agarwal A. *Illustrative Guide to Cataract Surgery: A Step-by-Step Approach to Refining Surgical Skills*. Thorofare, NJ: SLACK Incorporated; 2012.)

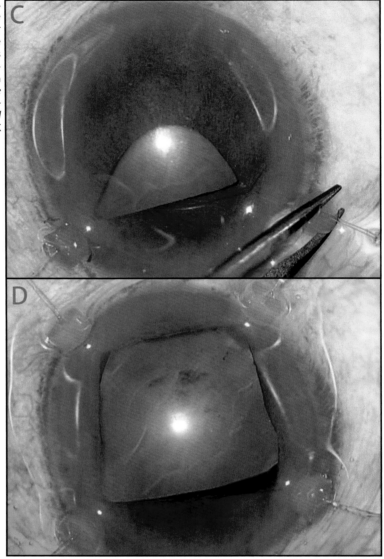

configuration for phacoemulsification.[9] He developed metal iris retractors connected to small blocks of titanium. The latter allows for stabilization of the hooks during the retraction of the iris. De Juan and Hickingbotham[10] enhanced this method with the introduction of the flexible iris retractor.

Traditionally, 4 evenly spaced retractors are placed through limbal paracenteses 90 degrees apart from one another. The corneal incision is centered on 1 of the 4 sides of the square. The "diamond configuration" of iris hook placement was first suggested by Dr. Thomas Oetting,[11] with one of the hooks located subincisionally, which helps prevent IFIS syndrome.

The iris hook may catch and damage the capsule during engagement with the pupillary edge, leading to an anterior capsule tear that may extend to the periphery. To avoid this problem, a drop of viscoelastic material should be injected between the iris and the capsule before the hook is inserted. Another useful technique is to keep the hook parallel to the iris plane during insertion

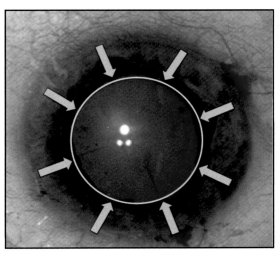

Figure 3-3. Eight-point iris margin fixation is achieved with the Malyugin ring, providing perfectly round pupillary aperture.

and to slightly tilt it posteriorly near the pupillary edge to engage the iris only. Iris hooks may become loosened during surgery and may become dislocated, no longer holding the pupillary edge. This can cause problems, including iris aspiration and chafing from contact with the phacoemulsification needle.

Pupil Expansion Rings

The following pupil expansion devices currently in the market include:

- Graether pupil expander (Eagle Vision, Memphis, TN)
- Siepser ring
- Perfect Pupil (Milvella Limited, North Sydney, New South Wales, Australia)
- Morcher ring (Morcher GmbH, Stuttgart, Germany)
- Oasis Ring (Oasis Medical, Glendora, CA)

Malyugin Ring

The Malyugin ring (MicroSurgical Technology, Redmond, WA) is a pupil expansion device made of 5-0 polypropylene with a square shape and 4 equidistantly located circular loops. The loop at each angle has a wedge-shaped gap facing outward and is designed to accommodate the iris tissue. One of the main advantages of this device is that it has 8 points of fixation of the iris tissue. As a result of omnidirectional stretching—and in spite of the fact that the ring has a square shape—the expanded pupil looks round after implantation of the Malyugin ring (Figure 3-3).

The Malyugin ring is available in 2 sizes: 6.25 mm and 7.0 mm. The advantage of the smaller ring is that it is easier to insert and to retract. The 7.0-mm ring provides larger exposure of the lens nucleus and is preferable for the surgeon using a phaco flip nucleus removal technique. Complete evacuation of the cortical material with the 7.0-mm Malyugin ring can be easier.

The Malyugin ring system consists of a presterilized, single-use holder containing the ring and the inserter (Figure 3-4). The ring is usually inserted at the beginning of the phaco procedure through an unenlarged 1.8- to 2.8-mm clear corneal incision into the pupillary aperture. The ring is injected while simultaneously retracting the injector. Capsulorrhexis, hydrodissection, phacoemulsification, and injection of the intraocular lens (IOL) are performed through the expanded pupil with the device in place. In the event of necessity (progressive intraoperative pupil constriction), the ring can be inserted at any stage of the surgical procedure.

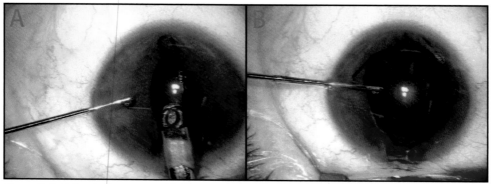

Figure 3-4. Malyugin ring system. (A) The insertion of the Malyugin ring is carried out through the main incision with the help of an injector. (B) With the Malyugin ring in place, the pupil is sufficiently expanded to provide adequate surgical exposure.

The technique of the Malyugin ring insertion and removal is variable, depending on the size of the incision. With a 2.2-mm and larger incision, the inserter can pass through the corneal tunnel into the anterior chamber (Figure 3-5). After lens removal and IOL implantation, the proximal and distant ring scrolls are disengaged from the pupillary margin one by one. The injector is inserted through the main incision to catch the proximal ring scroll and retract the device from the eye.

Malyugin Ring in Posterior Capsular Rupture

Agarwal et al[3] modified the technique for using the Malyugin ring to ensure safe iris expansion in small pupil cataract surgery in eyes with posterior capsule defects. In this method, a 6-0 polyglactin suture is placed in the leading scroll of the Malyugin ring and injected into the pupillary plane (Figure 3-6). The end of the suture remains at the main incision. Once in place, the ring produces a stable mydriasis of approximately 6.0 mm. Thereby, an IOL can be implanted easily in the sulcus with visualization, which prevents the inadvertent dropping of the iris expander into the vitreous during intraoperative manipulation. This modification has 2 main advantages. First, the ring dropping into the vitreous due to poor capsule support is reduced as it is well secured by the suture. Second, if a large posterior capsule defect occurs and the ring slips into the vitreous, it can be pulled back easily with the suture end. Thus, the surgeon can work effectively below the pupillary plane without fear of the ring slipping into the vitreous.

CONCLUSION

Different techniques of nucleus disassembly in small-incision cataract surgery require a wide and unobstructed view of the anterior portion of the lens, as well as the instruments, inserted into the anterior chamber. A well-dilated pupil helps to prevent the occurrence of posterior capsular rupture.

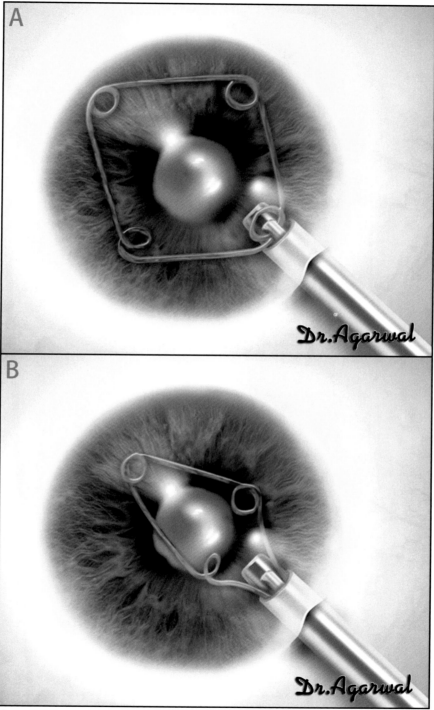

Figure 3-5. Removal of the Malyugin ring. (A) The injector is introduced into the anterior chamber and the trailing scroll is engaged by first sliding the thumb distally and then proximally. (B) Once the scroll is engaged, the thumb is slid distally to pull the scroll into the injector. The injector with the used Malyugin ring inside is then withdrawn from the eye. (Reprinted with permission from Agarwal A. *Illustrative Guide to Cataract Surgery: A Step-by-Step Approach to Refining Surgical Skills.* Thorofare, NJ: SLACK Incorporated; 2012.)

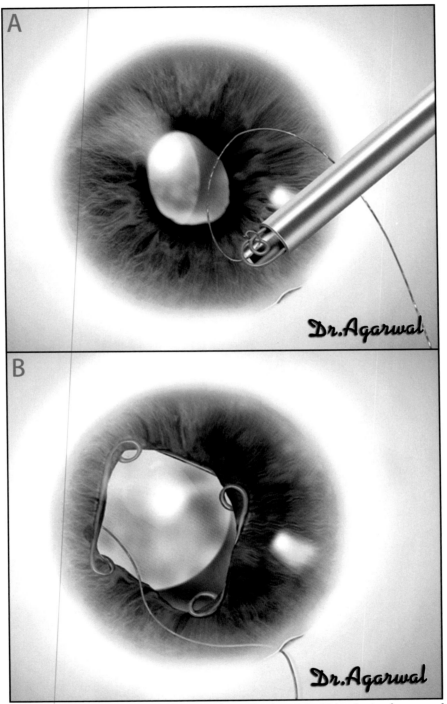

Figure 3-6. Illustration depicting the Agarwal modification of the Malyugin ring for cases of small pupil with a posterior capsular rupture. (A) A 6-0 suture is tied to the ring. (B) Malyugin ring is placed in the pupil. The suture can be pulled tighter if the ring begins to fall into the vitreous. (Reprinted with permission from Agarwal A. *Illustrative Guide to Cataract Surgery: A Step-by-Step Approach to Refining Surgical Skills.* Thorofare, NJ: SLACK Incorporated; 2012.)

REFERENCES

1. Malyugin B. Small pupil phaco surgery: a new technique. *Ann Ophthalmol.* 2007;39(3):185-193.
2. Chang D. Use of Malyugin pupil expansion device for intraoperative floppy-iris syndrome: results in 30 consecutive cases. *J Cataract Refract Surg.* 2008;34(5):835-841.
3. Agarwal A, Malyugin B, Kumar DA, et al. Modified Malyugin ring iris expansion technique in small-pupil cataract surgery with posterior capsule defect. *J Cataract Refract Surg.* 2008;34:724-726.
4. Malyugin B. Review of surgical management of small pupils in cataract surgery. Use of the Malyugin ring. *Techniques in Ophthalmology.* 2010;8(3):1-15.
5. Malyugin B. The new iris management technique in small pupil cataract surgery. In: Albert DM, Lucarelli MJ, eds. *Clinical Atlas of Procedures in Ophthalmic Surgery.* Chicago, IL: American Medical Association; 2011:18-26.
6. Malyugin B. Pupil issues in cataract surgery. *Cataract and Refractive Surgery Today.* 2012;(4):1-3.
7. Chang DF, Campbell JR. Intraoperative floppy iris syndrome associated with tamsulosin. *J Cataract Refract Surg.* 2005;31(4):664-673.
8. Miller KM, Keener GT Jr. Stretch pupilloplasty for small pupil phacoemulsification. *Am J Ophthalmol.* 1994;117:107-108.
9. Mackool RJ. Small pupil enlargement during cataract extraction. A new method. *J Cataract Refract Surg.* 1992;18(5):523-526.
10. de Juan E Jr, Hickingbotham D. Flexible iris retractor. *Am J Ophthalmol.* 1991;111(6):776-777.
11. Oetting TA, Omphroy LC. Modified technique using flexible iris retractors in clear corneal cataract surgery. *J Cataract Refract Surg.* 2002;28(4):596-598.

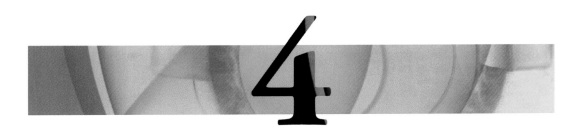

Posterior Polar Cataracts

Abhay R. Vasavada, MS, FRCS and Shetal M. Raj, MS

Posterior polar cataract (PPC) is a clinically distinctive entity consisting of a dense, white, well demarcated, disk-shaped opacity located in the posterior cortex or subcapsular region. Two types of PPC, stationary and progressive, have been described in literature.[1] The stationary type consists of concentric rings around the central plaque opacity that looks like a bullseye (Figure 4-1). This type is compatible with good vision. Usually, the patient seeks medical help in the third or the fourth decade of life. The most common symptom is intolerance to light. Glare is most severe when the light source is close to the object of vision. In the progressive type, changes occur in the posterior cortex in the form of radiating rider opacities. Patients with progressive opacity become more symptomatic as the peripheral extensions enlarge.

The inheritance pattern of PPC is reported to be autosomal dominant.[2-7] Osher et al[8] reported a positive family history for congenital cataracts in 55% (12 of 22) of patients. The gene for PPC has been linked with the haptoglobin locus on chromosome 16.[9] A recent study reported that mutations in the PITX3 gene in humans results in PPC and variable anterior segment mesenchymal dysgenesis.[10] Previous studies have indicated that a majority of such patients present with bilateral cataracts; the incidence being 80% as reported in the authors' earlier study[11] and 70% reported in a study by Gavris et al.[12] There is no gender predilection in PPC. The polar opacity consists of abnormal lens fiber cells and an accumulation of extracellular materials.[13-15]

PPC presents a special challenge to the phacoemulsification surgeon, as it is known to be predisposed to posterior capsule dehiscence during surgery.[8,11] In 1990, Osher et al[8] reported a 26% (8 of 31 eyes) incidence of posterior capsular rupture during surgery in eyes with PPC. In 1999, the authors reported a 36% (9 of 25 eyes) incidence,[11] whereas in 2003, Hayashi et al[16] and Lee and Lee[17] reported an incidence of 7.1% (2 of 28 eyes) and 11% (4 of 36 eyes), respectively. Liu et al[18] reported an incidence of 16.4% (10 of 61 eyes). A study by Gavris et al[12] in 2004 reported an incidence of 40% (4 of 10 eyes).

Agarwal A.
*Posterior Capsular Rupture: A Practical Guide
to Prevention and Management* (pp 41-49).
© 2014 Taylor & Francis Group.

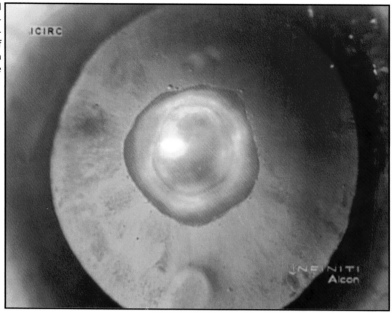

Figure 4-1. PPC characterized by dense, white, well demarcated, disk-shaped opacity. In the stationary type of PPC, concentric rings are seen around the central plaque opacity resembling a bullseye.

To prevent posterior capsular rupture, Osher et al[8] recommends slow-motion phacoemulsification with low aspiration flow rate (AFR), vacuum, and infusion pressure. Fine et al[19] avoided overpressurization of the anterior chamber with viscodissection to mobilize the epinucleus and cortex, Allen and Wood[20] also performed viscodissection, and Lee and Lee[17] preferred a lambda technique with dry aspiration. The authors prefer inside-out delineation.[21] This technique, along with modern instrumentation, refined surgical strategies, and better understanding of phacodynamics and cumulative surgical experience has enabled us to reduce the incidence of posterior capsular rupture to 8% (2 of 25 eyes).[21]

DIAGNOSIS

A bullseye appearance is pathognomonic of PPC. However, this entity could be camouflaged under a dense nuclear sclerosis or a total white cataract. In the authors' opinion, surgery should be delayed as long as possible and should be undertaken only if the patient finds it difficult to perform his or her routine activities. In the authors' experience, the procedure should be governed by the following paradigm.

SURGICAL TECHNIQUE

Counseling

During preoperative examination, the patient should be informed of the possibility of intraoperative posterior capsular rupture-related dropped nucleus, relatively longer operative time, secondary posterior segment intervention, and likely delay of visual recovery. The need to perform neodymium-doped yttrium aluminum garnet (Nd:YAG) capsulotomy for residual plaque[8,11,16] and the possibility of preexisting amblyopia, especially in unilateral PPC, should be envisaged at the preliminary stage.[16]

Anesthesia

Peribulbar anesthesia with oculopressure to soften the globe diminishes intraoperative posterior pressure.[8] With increasing experience, the surgeon may use topical anesthesia in a selective manner.

Surgical Technique

The authors prefer to use a closed chamber technique. The contours of the cornea and the globe should be maintained throughout the procedure.

Hayashi et al[16] performs either phacoemulsification, pars plana lensectomy, or intracapsular cataract extraction, depending on the size of the opacity and the density of nuclear sclerosis.

Incision

A paracentesis is performed with a 15-degree ophthalmic knife. The aqueous is exchanged with sodium hyaluronate (Provisc). A temporal corneal, single-plane valvular incision of 2.6 mm is performed. A cohesive viscoelastic in the anterior chamber prevents chamber collapse and forward movement of iris-lens diaphragm during entry into the eye. Fine et al[19] cautioned against increasing the pressure in the anterior chamber.

Capsulorrhexis

The optimal capsulorrhexis size is approximately ≤5 mm. Although a rhexis size of ≤4 mm could be detrimental in the event of necessity to prolapse the nucleus into the anterior chamber, a larger opening may not leave adequate support for a sulcus-fixated intraocular lens (IOL) in the event the posterior chamber is compromised.[11,19]

Hydro Procedures

Cortico-cleaving hydrodissection,[22] can lead to hydraulic rupture and should be avoided.[8,11] It would be logical to perform hydrodelineation to create a mechanical cushion of epinucleus.[11,16,20,23] Masket,[24] Hayashi et al,[16] Allen and Wood,[20] and Lee and Lee[17] recommended hydrodelineation. In addition to hydrodelineation, Fine et al[19] also performs hydrodissection in multiple quadrants, injecting tiny amounts of fluid gently, such that the fluid wave is not allowed to spread and extend across the posterior capsule.

The authors propose inside-out delineation to precisely delineate the central core of nucleus.[21]

Inside-Out Delineation

A central trench is sculpted with the slow motion technique in the Infinity Vision System (Alcon Laboratories, Fort Worth, TX). In nuclear sclerosis ≤Grade 3 (grading system from Grade 1 to 5),[25] preset parameters are ultrasound (US) energy 30% to 60% (supraoptimal power), vacuum 60 mm Hg, AFR 18 cc/min, and bottle height (BH) 70 cm. Care should be taken not to mechanically rock the lens. Dispersive viscoelastic (Viscoat) is injected through the sideport before retracting the probe to avoid forward movement of iris-lens diaphragm. A specially designed, right-angled cannula mounted on a 2-cc syringe filled with fluid is introduced through the main incision, and the tip is placed adjacent to the right wall of the trench at an appropriate depth, depending on the density of the cataract. It then penetrates the central lens substance, and fluid is injected through the right wall of the trench (Figure 4-2). Delineation is produced by the fluid traversing inside-out. A golden ring within the lens is evidence of successful delineation (Figure 4-3). Fluid injection may be repeated in the left wall of the trench with another right-angled cannula (Figure 4-4). The trench allows the surgeon to reach the central core of the nucleus. As fluid is injected at a desired depth under direct vision, a desired thickness of epinucleus cushion can be achieved. It provides a

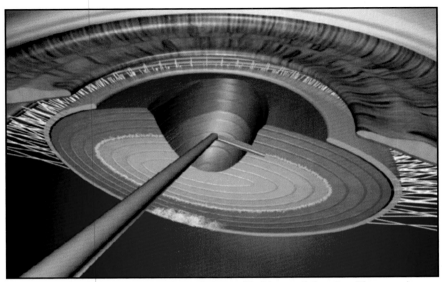

Figure 4-2. Sketch demonstrating the technique of inside-out delineation. The cannula penetrates the central lens substance and fluid is injected through the right wall of the trench.

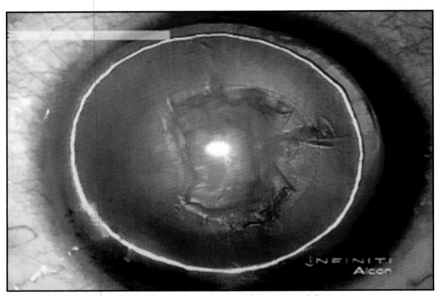

Figure 4-3. The golden ring indicates the end point of inside-out delineation.

precise epinucleus bowl that acts as a mechanical cushion to protect the posterior capsule during subsequent maneuvers.

With conventional hydrodelineation, the cannula is penetrated within the lens substance causing the fluid to traverse from outside to inside. It is sometimes difficult to introduce the cannula within a firm nucleus, which leads to rocking and stress on the capsular bag and zonules. There is also a possibility of fluid being inadvertently injected into the subcapsular plane, leading to unwarranted hydrodissection. Inside-out delineation is easy to perform, provides superior control, reduces stress to zonules, and precisely demarcates the central core of nucleus.

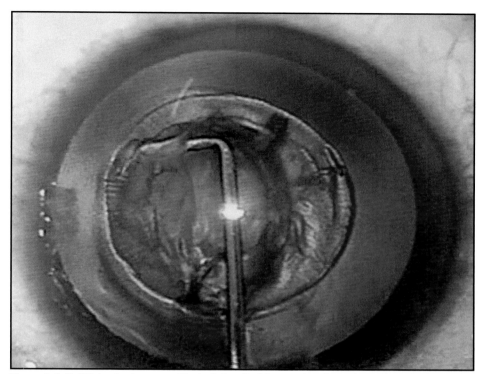

Figure 4-4. Fluid injection is repeated in the left wall of the trench with another right-angled cannula if delineation is incomplete.

Rotation

Any attempt to rotate the nucleus can lead to posterior capsular rupture and is therefore avoided.[11]

Division and Fragment Removal

All techniques that are geared to facilitate the removal of nucleus within the cushion affect the epinucleus. Bimanual cracking and division of the nucleus involve outward movements and can result in distortion of the capsular bag. In nuclear sclerosis ≥2 the authors use the step-by-step chop in situ and lateral separation technique[26]; for chopping, use US 40% to 50%, vacuum 150 to 250 mm Hg, AFR 18 cc/min, and BH 70 to 90 cm. The resultant fragments are removed with the stop, chop, chop and stuff technique.[27] In nuclear sclerosis <2, the entire nucleus is aspirated within the epinucleus shell using AFR 16 cc/min and vacuum 100 to 120 mm Hg. Figure 4-5 shows the capsular bag after nucleus removal and shows a central breach in the continuity of the epinucleus at the site of the PPC. Traction of posterior lens fibers and posterior polar opacity during surgery are enough to break the weak posterior capsule. Thus, the slow-motion technique is recommended to reduce turbulence in the anterior chamber.[28] Collapse of the anterior chamber and forward bulge of the posterior chamber is prevented throughout the procedure by injecting viscoelastic before the instrument is withdrawn.[11,29]

Lee and Lee[17] use the lambda technique to sculpt the nucleus, followed by cracking along both arms and removal of central piece.

Figure 4-5. Capsular bag after nucleus removal, showing a central breach in the continuity of epinucleus at the site of the PPC.

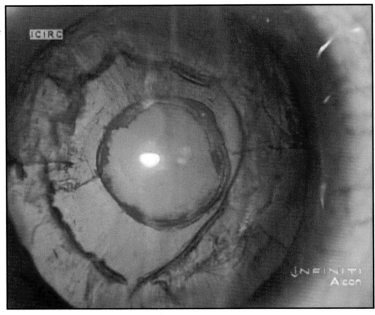

Figure 4-6. Sketch demonstrating the technique of injecting fluid in the subcapsular region to cleave the cortex from the capsule proximal to the incision. The nucleus has been emulsified and the capsular bag is empty. Therefore, it is safe to hydrodissect at this stage.

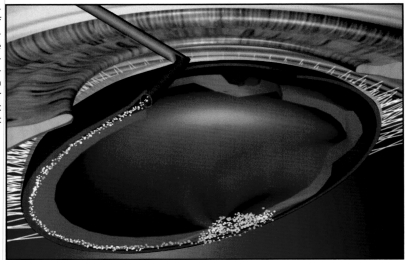

Epinucleus Removal

First, only the peripheral lower half of epinucleus is stripped off using US 30%, vacuum 80 to 100 mm Hg, AFR 16 cc/min, and BH 80 to 90 cm. The central area is left attached.[11,19,24] Then, the peripheral upper epinucleus (subincisional epinucleus) is mobilized with a gentle focal and multiquadrant hydrodissection with a right-angled cannula facing right and left (Figure 4-6). The fluid wave travels along the cleavage formed between the capsule and the lower epinucleus, which does not threaten the integrity of the posterior capsule. It is safe to hydrodissect because the capsular bag is not fully occupied. Therefore, the hydraulic pressure that is built up is not sufficient to rupture the posterior capsule. The entire epinucleus is then aspirated, finally detaching the central area.

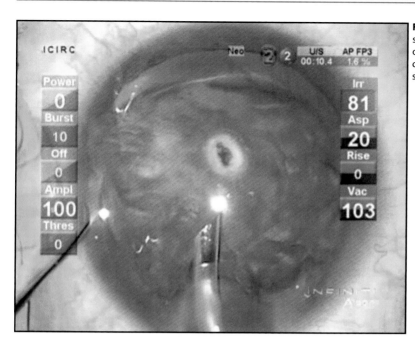

Figure 4-7. A pseudohole suggestive of a defect is observed in the posterior cortex, but the posterior capsule remains intact.

Fine et al[19] and Allen and Wood[20] suggest that viscodissection of the epinucleus be performed by injecting viscoelastic (Healon 5 or Healon GV and Viscoat) under the capsular edge to mobilize the rim of epinucleus. It is removed with a coaxial irrigation/aspiration (I/A) handpiece. Lee and Lee[17] performed manual dry aspiration with a Simcoe cannula.

Pseudohole

At times, the classical appearance suggestive of a defect is observed in the posterior cortex, but the posterior capsule remains intact. This is a known as a *pseudohole* (Figure 4-7).

Cortex Removal

Bimanual automated I/A, using AFR 20 cc/min and vacuum 400 mm Hg, optimizes control, ensures anterior chamber maintenance, and aids in the complete removal of the cortex. Fine et al[19] used coaxial I/A to protect the posterior chamber during cortex removal.

Posterior Capsule Vacuum Polishing

Posterior capsule vacuum polishing is avoided even if the posterior chamber is not open because of its potential fragility.[8,11,16,19,24] The traction on an excessively adhered plaque to an otherwise normal posterior capsule could eventually rupture the posterior capsule. Instead, postoperative Nd:YAG laser posterior capsulotomy is preferable.

POSTERIOR CAPSULE DEHISCENCE

If a defect is present in the posterior chamber, Viscoat is injected over the area of the posterior chamber defect before the phaco or I/A probe is withdrawn from the eye,[29] and 2-port limbal anterior vitrectomy is performed using a cut rate of 800 cuts/min, vacuum 300 mm Hg, and AFR

25 cc/min. Once the anterior chamber is free from vitreous, the cortex is aspirated by bimanual I/A. A posterior continuous curvilinear capsulorrhexis (PCCC) may be performed if the rupture is confined to a small central area.

Intraocular Lens Implantation

In eyes with posterior chamber defect, the IOL is implanted in the bag only if PCCC can be achieved. In eyes with a large posterior capsule defect, the IOL is placed over the anterior capsule in the ciliary sulcus. Fine et al[19] and Gimbel and DeBroff[30] have suggested capture of the optic through the anterior capsulorrhexis. The authors believe that optic capture induces more inflammation.[31]

After IOL implantation, viscoelastic is removed by a 2-port vitrectomy, rather than I/A, as vitrectomy aspirates in a piecemeal and gradual manner and reduces the chances of rapid aspiration of vitreous.

The authors do not suture the main valvular incision, but do suture the paracentesis in eyes with posterior capsule defect. In such eyes, a periodic evaluation for retinal break, cystoid macular edema, and raised intraocular pressure is necessary.

SURGICAL PEARLS

- Thorough counseling during preoperative work-up avoids patient dissatisfaction postoperatively.
- Cortico-cleaving hydrodissection should be avoided as it increases the risk of posterior capsule dehiscence.
- Inside-out delineation will effectively delineate the nucleus from the epinucleus shell.
- Adhering to the principles of closed chamber technique throughout the surgery prevents sudden collapse of the anterior chamber with anterior movement of the iris-lens diaphragm.
- The slow-motion technique for lens removal reduces turbulence in the eye.
- Focal and multiquadrant hydrodissection effectively cleaves the subincisional epinucleus.

REFERENCES

1. Duke-Elder S. Posterior polar cataract. In: Duke-Elder S, ed. *System of Ophthalmology: Normal and Abnormal Development, Congenital Deformities.* Vol 3, Pt 2. St Louis, MO: CV Mosby; 1964:723-726.
2. Tulloh CG. Hereditary posterior polar cataract with report of a pedigree. *Br J Ophthalmol.* 1955;39(6):374-379.
3. Tulloh CG. Hereditary posterior polar cataract. *Br J Ophthalmol.* 1956;40(9):566-567.
4. Nettleship E, Ogilvie FM. A peculiar form of hereditary congenital cataract. *Trans Ophthalmol Soc UK.* 1906;26:191-207.
5. Harman NB. New pedigree of cataract—posterior polar, anterior polar and microphthalmia, and lamellar. *Trans Ophthalmol Soc UK.* 1909;29:296-306.
6. Yamada K, Tomita HA, Kanazawa S, Mera A, Amemiya T, Niikawa N. Genetically distinct autosomal dominant posterior polar cataract in a four-generation Japanese family. *Am J Ophthalmol.* 2000;129(2):159-165.
7. Berry V, Francis P, Reddy MA, et al. Alpha-B crystallin gene (CRYAB) mutation causes dominant congenital posterior polar cataract in humans. *Am J Hum Genet.* 2001;69(5):1141-1145.
8. Osher RH, Yu BC, Koch DD. Posterior polar cataracts: a predisposition to intraoperative posterior capsular rupture. *J Cataract Refract Surg.* 1990;16:157-162.
9. Maumenee IH. Classification of hereditary cataracts in children by linkage analysis. Ophthalmology. 1979;86:1554-1558.

10. Addison PK, Berry V, Ionides AC, Francis PJ, Bhattacharya SS, Moore AT. Posterior polar cataract is the predominant consequence of a recurrent mutation in the PITX3 gene. *Br J Ophthalmol.* 2005;89(2):138-141.

11. Vasavada AR, Singh R. Phacoemulsification with posterior polar cataract. *J Cataract Refract Surg.* 1999;25:238-245.

12. Gavris M, Popa D, Caraus C, et al. Phacoemulsification in posterior polar cataract. *Oftalmologia.* 2004;48(4):36-40.

13. Eshaghian J, Streeten BW. Human posterior subcapsular cataract; an ultrastructural study of the posteriorly migrating cells. *Arch Ophthalmol.* 1980;98:134-143.

14. Eshagian J. Human posterior subcapsular cataracts. *Trans Ophthalmol Soc UK.* 1982;102:364-368.

15. Nagata M, Marsuura H, Fujinaga Y. Ultrastructure of posterior subcapsular cataract in human lens. *Ophthalmic Res.* 1986;18:180-184.

16. Hayashi K, Hayashi H, Nakao F, et al. Outcomes of surgery for posterior polar cataract. *J Cataract Refract Surg.* 2003;29:45-49.

17. Lee MW, Lee YC. Phacoemulsification of posterior polar cataracts: a surgical challenge. *Br J Ophthalmol.* 2003;87:1426-1427.

18. Liu Y, Liu Y, Wu M, Zhang X. Phacoemulsification in eyes with posterior polar cataract and foldable intraocular lens implantation. *Yan Ke Xue Bao.* 2003;19(2):92-94.

19. Fine IH, Packer M, Hoffman RS. Management of posterior polar cataract. *J Cataract Refract Surg.* 2003;29:16-19.

20. Allen D, Wood C. Minimizing risk to the capsule during surgery for posterior polar cataract. *J Cataract Refract Surg.* 2002;28:742-744.

21. Vasavada AR, Raj SM. Inside-out delineation. *J Cataract Refract Surg.* 2004;30:1167-1169.

22. Fine IH. Cortico-cleaving hydrodissection. *J Cataract Refract Surg.* 1992;18:508-512.

23. Anis AY. Understanding hydrodelineation: the term and procedure. *Doc Ophthalmol.* 1994;87(2):123-137.

24. Masket S. Cataract surgical problem. Consultation section. *J Cataract Refract Surg.* 1997;23:819-824.

25. Emery JM, Little JH. *Phacoemulsification and Aspiration of Cataracts, Surgical Technique, Complications and Results.* St Louis, MO: CV Mosby; 1979:45-49.

26. Vasavada AR, Singh R. Step-by-step chop in situ and separation of very dense cataracts. *J Cataract Refract Surg.* 1998;24:156-159.

27. Vasavada AR, Desai JP. Stop, chop, chop and stuff. *J Cataract Refract Surg.* 1996;22:526-529.

28. Osher RH. Slow motion phacoemulsification approach (letter). *J Cataract Refract Surg.* 1993;19(5):667.

29. Osher RH, Cionni R. Intra-operative complications of phacoemulsification surgery. In: Steinert RF, ed. *Cataract Surgery: Techniques, Complications and Management.* 2nd ed. Philadelphia, PA: Saunders Elsevier; 2004:469-486.

30. Gimbel HV, DeBroff BM. Posterior capsulorhexis with optic capture: maintaining a clear visual axis after pediatric cataract surgery. *J Cataract Refract Surg.* 1994;20:658-664.

31. Vasavada AR, Trivedi R. Role of optic capture in congenital cataract and IOL surgery in children. *J Cataract Refract Surg.* 2000;26:824-831.

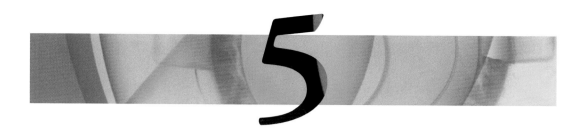

Subluxated Cataracts

Kevin M. Miller, MD and Amar Agarwal, MS, FRCS, FRCOphth

A lens is subluxated when it does not sit in the normal anatomic position with respect to the pupil (Figures 5-1 and 5-2). If the lens is completely dislocated into the anterior chamber or vitreous cavity, it is termed *luxation*. A subluxation is essentially a partial luxation.[1-15] It also goes by the name *ectopia lentis*. In this condition, the lens most often displaces laterally with respect to the pupil and the problem can be congenital or acquired. Alternatively and frequently, the lens can appear normal at birth but it can displace slowly and progressively over subsequent years. Most ophthalmologists consider lens subluxation to be more difficult to manage surgically than diffuse zonular laxity or focal zonular loss without subluxation, but all of these conditions can be challenging.

POSTERIOR CAPSULAR RUPTURE

So, how does subluxation relate to posterior capsular rupture? There are several areas where the 2 entities intersect. First, zonular laxity, or dehiscence, increases the odds of posterior capsular rupture. Many subluxated cataracts are dense, so the odds of posterior capsular rupture increases (Figure 5-3). Second, any lack of zonular countertraction during surgery may lead to difficulty with phacoemulsification, cortex removal, and device implantation. Finally, zonular laxity, which always accompanies lens subluxation, makes it more difficult to manage a posterior capsular rupture after it occurs.

DISCERNING THE EXTENT OF ZONULAR WEAKNESS

It is important for the ophthalmologist to detect zonular weakness before taking a patient to the operating room. The zonulopathy will almost always appear worse under the operating

Agarwal A.
Posterior Capsular Rupture: A Practical Guide to Prevention and Management (pp 51-67).
© 2014 Taylor & Francis Group.

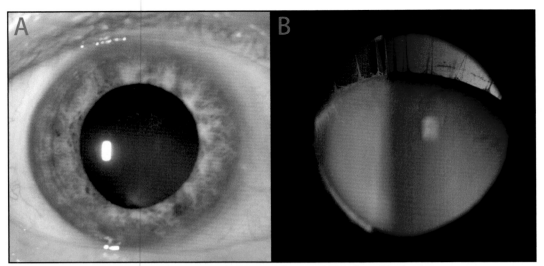

Figure 5-1. An inferiorly subluxated cataract is shown in (A) direct and (B) indirect illumination.

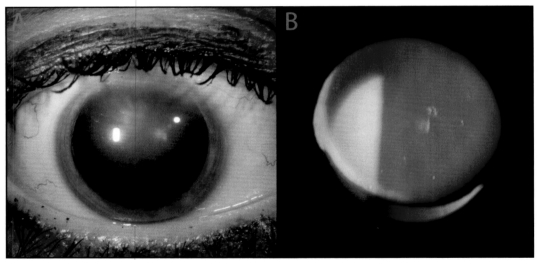

Figure 5-2. A superiorly subluxated cataract is shown in (A) direct and (B) indirect illumination.

microscope than it did at the slit-lamp biomicroscope. Subluxation does not accompany every case of zonular weakness; it appears only in advanced cases. What is the best way to detect a zonulopathy? It is best identified at the slit-lamp biomicroscope. The signs are occasionally obvious, but more often than not they are subtle.

Beginning ophthalmologists often ask their patients to look from side to side while they observe for lens jiggle at the precise moment the eyes stop moving. However, this can be difficult to see. Some ophthalmologists pound their fist against the table on which the slit-lamp biomicroscope is sitting and look for lens movement. The authors are not a big fan of this approach, as it is uncomfortable for the patient. Experienced ophthalmologists become good at detecting the inevitable microsaccades that occur whenever a patient attempts to maintain fixation. Although subtle, these microsaccades have high angular velocities and produce some of the most easily detectable lens movements. Finally, iridodonesis often occurs in the presence of phacodonesis. If iridodonesis is seen, it should tip off the ophthalmologist to look for phacodonesis. Phacodonesis can be detected

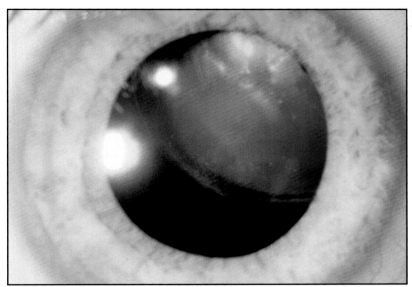

Figure 5-3. Dense dislocated cataract.

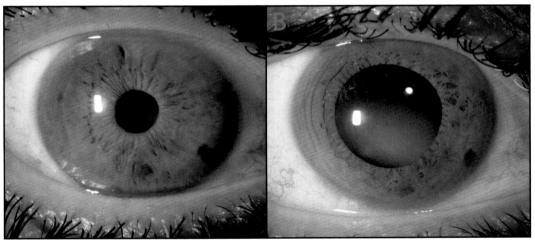

Figure 5-4. (A) This middle-aged man complained of unstable vision. He had narrow angle configuration and had undergone laser peripheral iridotomies in both eyes. (B) Mild phacodonesis was present before dilation, and prominent phacodonesis was evident after dilation. Dilation also revealed inferior subluxation in both eyes.

with the pupil undilated or dilated, but it is usually easier to see when the pupil is dilated. With dilation, there is less iris tissue available to stabilize the anterior lens capsule (Figure 5-4). In addition, if a subluxation is present, good dilation will expose it.

Lens subluxation occurs in the setting of profound diffuse zonular weakness. The zonules on one side of the lens are weaker than the zonules on the other side, leading to lens movement in the direction of the stronger zonules. If all zonules are diffusely and profoundly lax, a sunset syndrome results, whereby the lens sinks by gravity into the anterior portion of the posterior segment.

Some lenses are perfectly centered behind the pupil, yet careful inspection at the time of surgery reveals that the zonules spanning one or more clock hours are damaged or absent. In such cases, the remaining zonules maybe strong, but the odds are substantial that there is diffuse damage to all the zonules.

Figure 5-5. This older man suffered blunt trauma to his right eye many years earlier. He presented with a mature white cataract and an indentation of the lens equator adjacent to the area of zonular dehiscence.

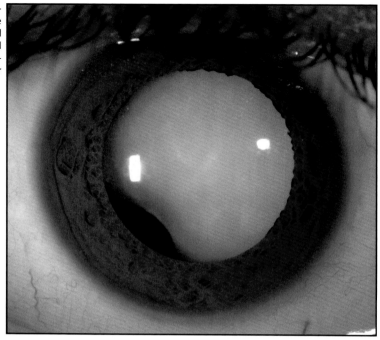

Certain clinical findings can alert the observer as to the relative age of the zonular defects. Segmental defects that are relatively new may be difficult to identify unless there is vitreous prolapse around the lens equator or a clear-cut surgical history. Older defects, however, may be associated with a flattening or indentation of the lens equator. This is often known as a *lens coloboma*, although the term is inaccurate because there is no actual loss of lens tissue (Figure 5-5).

Conditions Associated With Phacodonesis and Lens Subluxation

A number of ocular and systemic conditions are associated with phacodonesis and subluxation, some of which are causative. It is important to verify the significant associations because of the potential for early diagnosis and medical or surgical intervention in these conditions. Often, there is a progression from focal zonular dehiscence to diffuse zonular laxity to phacodonesis to lens subluxation, so the authors think it is best to consider these entities on a continuum, rather than as discrete categories.

In Dr. Miller's practice, the most common cause of zonulopathy is ocular trauma. The zonulopathy is only one problem among many that the trauma causes (Figure 5-6). The second most common cause of zonulopathy is pseudoexfoliation syndrome. The third most common cause, interestingly, is idiopathic. Many eyes have zonular weakness and evidence of mild phacodonesis, with no evidence of ocular or systemic comorbidity. Some of these eyes may be early cases of pseudoexfoliation syndrome, but they do not manifest pupillary border transillumination defects or evidence of pseudoexfoliation changes in the fellow eye. Many other conditions exist as well. Systemic conditions include Marfan syndrome, homocystinuria, and Ehlers-Danlos syndrome. Ocular conditions include retinopathy of prematurity, choroidal and ciliary body colobomas, and retinitis pigmentosa.

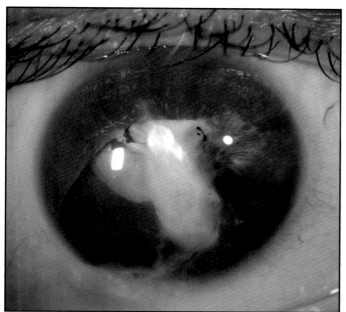

Figure 5-6. This man suffered a penetrating wire injury to his right eye when he was a child. In addition to an involuted and subluxated cataract, he suffered from a central corneal scar and iris tissue loss.

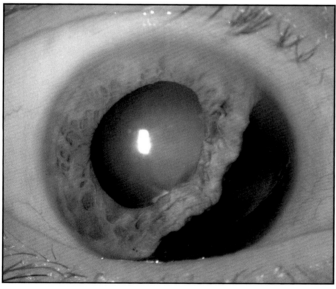

Figure 5-7. This man has a dense posterior subcapsular cataract and a large inferonasal iridodialysis following blunt eye trauma.

IDENTIFYING ASSOCIATED OCULAR COMORBIDITIES

In addition to finding ocular and systemic conditions that may be related etiologically to phacodonesis and lens subluxation, it is also important to identify associated ocular comorbidities. Surgical intervention of these conditions may be necessary at the time of cataract surgery. The patient should be counseled about the ramifications of his or her comorbidities on the likely visual outcome of surgery.

Associated conditions may include corneal scars, pupillary defects, iridodialysis (Figure 5-7), glaucoma, macular scars, cystoid macular edema, reduced visual potential, peripheral retinal pathology, visual field loss, and optic atrophy.

As an example, trauma may be associated with any or all of the aforementioned associated conditions. Pseudoexfoliation may be associated with glaucoma, visual field loss, and optic atrophy. Retinopathy of prematurity may be associated with glaucoma, macular scarring, reduced visual potential, peripheral retinal pathology, visual field loss, and optic atrophy. Retinitis pigmentosa may be associated with cystoid macular edema, reduced visual potential, and visual field loss. Choroidal and ciliary body colobomas may be associated with reduced visual potential, visual field loss, and optic atrophy.

POTENTIAL INTRAOPERATIVE PROBLEMS

If an ophthalmologist does not identify zonular laxity at the slit-lamp biomicroscope before surgery, there are several intraoperative cues that should be apparent. The first finding is evident at the time of the anterior capsulotomy. In the presence of diffuse zonular laxity, the cystotome will produce numerous anterior capsule striae as it punctures the anterior capsule. Next, the entire lens will follow as the capsulorrhexis is being torn because of a lack of zonular countertraction. During cataract removal, there will be more phacodonesis than usual. After the capsular bag is cleaned of cortex, it will also be floppy.

Several intraoperative problems exist that the ophthalmologist must be prepared to handle. They include vitreous prolapse and loss, iatrogenic weakening of additional zonules, loss of lens fragments around the equator of the lens, difficulty removing cortex, difficulty inserting capsular bag support devices, and difficulty inserting an intraocular lens (IOL).

Problems with vitreous prolapse can be reduced or treated by injecting a dispersive viscoelastic over the area of zonular dehiscence. If diffuse zonular laxity is present, a dispersive viscoelastic can be layered over the zonules for their full 360-degree extent. Crystalline lenses that are initially decentered with respect to the pupil will often become more centered after the viscoelastic is injected into the eye. The surgeon must keep a watchful eye on the vitreous. If it incarcerates into a phacoemulsification or irrigation/aspiration (I/A) probe, the aspiration must be discontinued immediately to avoid tearing the retina. Additional dispersive viscoelastic can be injected into the anterior chamber at any time.

Care should be taken during the entire procedure to avoid weakening the zonules further. This is best accomplished by using the stronger zonules for countertraction. For instance, sculpting should be done from the area of strong zonules into the area of weak zonules. Cortex removal should be performed in a similar manner. A circumferential stripping action is often gentler than a radial stripping action, particularly when cortex is stripped out of the area of greatest zonular weakness.

Care must be taken when nuclear fragments are being removed so that the fragments cannot escape around the capsular equator into the vitreous cavity. If they drop, it is best to allow a retinal surgeon remove them at a later date.

When placing a capsular tension ring (CTR), it is important to inject the device toward the area of greatest zonular laxity. This puts the greatest stress on the strongest zonules. The authors like to lay the device into the bag for approximately 180 degrees before advancing it. In this way, the authors minimize the likelihood of the leading portion of the ring snagging on a fold in the capsular equator (Figure 5-8). If all the zonules are diffusely loose, it may be necessary to insert capsule tension segments and secure them to the sclera before inserting a CTR (Figure 5-9). It is advisable to use capsular hooks before inserting the endocapsular rings so as to give better stability to the capsular bag (Figures 5-10 and 5-11). Dr. Ike Ahmed designed the Ike segments (Morcher GmbH, Stuttgart, Germany), which can be used for small segments.

Inserting a lens implant can be very difficult in the setting of zonular laxity. Again, if one portion of the zonules is weaker than another, it is best to insert the leading haptic toward the direction of the greatest zonular laxity. It is generally easier to implant lenses with flexible haptics than

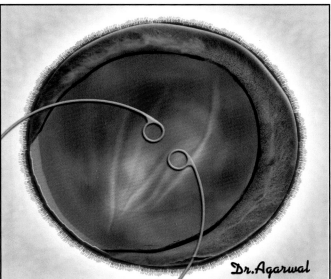

Figure 5-8. The endocapsular ring, or the CTR, can be inserted at any time during cataract surgery. It may also be implanted just prior to IOL insertion. It is advisable to insert capsular hooks as well at this stage to provide support to the bag during phaco maneuvers. (Reprinted with permission from Agarwal A. *Illustrative Guide to Cataract Surgery: A Step-by-Step Approach to Refining Surgical Skills.* Thorofare, NJ: SLACK Incorporated; 2012.)

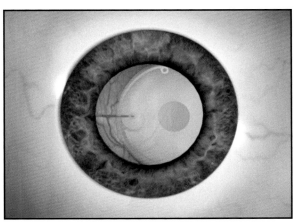

Figure 5-9. Cionni's ring. (Reprinted with permission from Dr. Agarwal's Eye Hospital, Chennai, India.)

lenses with stiff haptics. The trailing haptic can often be difficult to dial into a floppy capsular bag. Single-piece acrylic lenses are relatively easier to insert than 3-piece lenses with polymethyl methacrylate haptics.

POTENTIAL POSTOPERATIVE PROBLEMS

One may make it through cataract surgery successfully only to be plagued by a postoperative problem such as pseudophakodonesis or sunset syndrome. These problems can occur with or without a CTR in situ.

Pseudophakodonesis occurs as an early postoperative problem when there is diffuse zonular laxity. It may cause a patient to experience unstable vision or oscillopsia.

Sunset syndrome usually occurs as a late postoperative complication. As the name implies, the lens implant, along with entire capsular bag, slowly sinks into the pupil, eventually allowing the opacified anterior capsule to enter the pupillary space, followed sometime later by the equator of

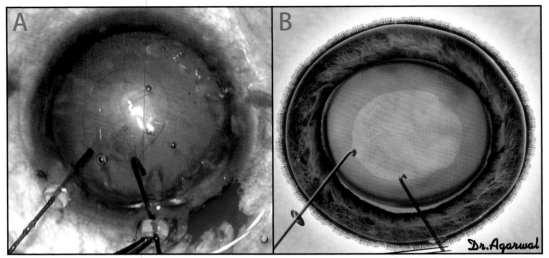

Figure 5-10. Capsular hooks are used in subluxated cataracts to support the capsular bag during phacoemulsification and other steps of cataract surgery. These are inserted through paracentesis wounds made at the limbus near the area of zonular dialysis. (Reprinted with permission from Agarwal A. *Illustrative Guide to Cataract Surgery: A Step-by-Step Approach to Refining Surgical Skills.* Thorofare, NJ: SLACK Incorporated; 2012.)

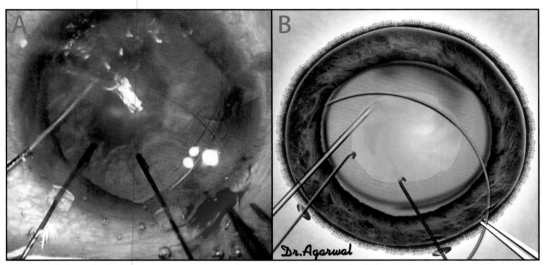

Figure 5-11. Capsular hooks are shown as they are hooked around the margin of the rhexis and they can be combined with insertion of a CTR as well for additional stability. They are removed at the end of surgery after insertion of the IOL. (Reprinted with permission from Agarwal A. *Illustrative Guide to Cataract Surgery: A Step-by-Step Approach to Refining Surgical Skills.* Thorofare, NJ: SLACK Incorporated; 2012.)

the IOL (Figure 5-12). Once this occurs, the patient experiences blurred vision and glare sensitivity. In advanced cases, the patient must look through an aphakic portion of the pupil.

INTRAOPERATIVE MANAGEMENT

Operating on patients with subluxated cataracts requires considerable planning and skill. The ophthalmologist must have all the necessary tools and devices available, as well as appropriate contingency plans should circumstances prevent the primary plan from being executed.

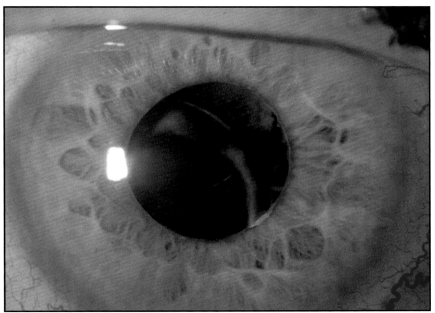

Figure 5-12. An older woman with severe pseudoexfoliation syndrome experienced a late dislocation of the capsular bag in her right eye. She experienced the same problem in her left eye years earlier and had undergone IOL exchange for an anterior chamber model, a complete capsulectomy, and anterior vitrectomy.

The surgeon should decide on the best anesthetic approach before arriving in the operating room. Topical anesthesia with intracameral supplementation should be avoided, as these surgeries are typically longer and require more intraoperative manipulation than can be successfully accomplished topically. For such cases, the author usually uses an orbital injection or general anesthesia.

The surgeon should decide ahead of time the best likely outcome. It may be an IOL inside the capsular bag, stabilized by a CTR alone. It may involve the addition of a capsule tension segment or a Cionni-modified CTR.[16] Scleral pockets will be necessary to fixate the device using the latter approach. The scleral pockets should be fashioned before the globe is entered. The authors' preference is for using Hoffman reverse scleral pockets. Appropriate suture material, either 9-0 Prolene or GORE-TEX, should be on hand. It is possible that the capsular bag will not be worth preserving and that the entire bag will have to be removed. In this scenario, an alternative method of lens fixation will have to be utilized. In the author's opinion, there is nothing wrong with an anterior chamber IOL if it is appropriately sized for the anterior chamber. Some surgeons prefer to suture fixate a lens to the posterior iris. Alternatively, a lens can be fixated to the sclera, either with sutures or by imbricating the haptics inside scleral tunnels, as in the glued IOL technique or the Scharioth technique.[17] Again, the surgeon should have a Plan A, as well as back-up Plans B and C.

After entering the anterior chamber, the surgeon should inject dispersive viscoelastic over any areas of the zonular dehiscence if the lens is subluxated and over the entire zonular apparatus if diffuse zonular laxity is present. The viscoelastic should be replaced as often as necessary to keep the vitreous back. Every effort should be made to establish a continuous tear capsulorrhexis. Radializing the capsular bag makes it difficult to stabilize the bag with hooks, should it become necessary.

A variety of capsular stabilization devices are available for intraoperative stabilization of the capsular bag during phacoemulsification and cortex removal. They should be inserted as early in the surgery as necessary to prevent further iatrogenic weakening of the zonules. If permanent fixation of the capsular bag is necessary, it may be more appropriate to implant capsular support devices early in the surgery and suture fixate them to the sclera.

Generally speaking, it is best to avoid implanting CTRs until as late in the surgery as absolutely necessary. Doing so early traps the cortex against the capsular equator and makes it more difficult to remove. The Henderson modification of the CTR makes this problem a little easier to handle.[16]

If a capsular bag is so flimsy that it collapses spontaneously on itself, the surgeon has to decide whether it is worth saving. The authors typically remove the capsular bag with a vitrector in such cases. There is simply no good argument for keeping a capsular bag in the eye when it collapses down to a 3- or 4-mm ball.

If the capsular bag can be preserved, a CTR should be implanted. Afterward, the lens epithelial cells lining the residual anterior capsule should be débrided with a pair of anterior capsule polishers. Doing so removes the cells that subsequently cause the capsular bag to shrink-wrap to the implant, adding additional stress to the zonules. By débriding the anterior capsule of these cells, the capsulorrhexis tends to stay open better after surgery, thereby avoiding the phimosis and lens implant decentration that may otherwise follow.

Although some surgeons advocate placing a lens in the ciliary sulcus and capturing the optic inside the capsular bag in the setting of diffuse zonular laxity, the authors have reservations that this may hasten the long-term demise of the zonules, making it more likely that the capsule will sunset. Doing so, however, does reduce the amount of pseudophakodonesis that is present shortly after surgery, as compared to in-the-bag implantation.

If an anterior vitrectomy becomes necessary, it should be performed bimanually with a high-speed cutter and a low-aspiration flow rate. If an anterior chamber lens implant becomes necessary, a good starting point for sizing the haptics is the horizontal corneal white-to-white dimension +1 mm. After the lens is in position within the anterior chamber, it should be inspected and replaced if it is too loose or too tight. A peripheral iridectomy should be fashioned before the incision is closed. The authors like to make the iridectomy with the vitrector prior to lens implantation.

It is relatively easy to tear the posterior capsule during phacoemulsification and CTR implantation, especially when the zonules are extremely weak. If the capsule tears, the author advocates removing the capsular bag in its entirety and proceeding with an alternate plan for lens implantation and fixation.

ASSIA CAPSULE ANCHOR

The Assia Capsule Anchor (AssiAnchor; Hanita Lenses, Kibbutz Hanita, Israel) is a novel device for managing subluxation of the lens associated with moderate to severe zonular dehiscence or weakness. This was designed by Dr. Ehud Assia from Israel. The Assia capsule anchor is a polymethyl methacrylate (PMMA) intraocular, uniplanar implant, inserted into the capsular bag after capsulorrhexis is performed. An intact anterior continuous curvilinear capsulorrhexis is a prerequisite for the safe use of the anchor. The 2 lateral arms of the device are inserted behind the anterior lens capsule, whereas the central rod is placed in front of the capsule (Figure 5-13). A 10-0, or preferably, a 9-0 Prolene suture is used to fixate the anchor to the scleral wall. The suture is either threaded through the hole in the base of the device or wrapped around the neck of the anterior rod. A temporary safety suture can be used to prevent the falling of the device through the large zonular defect during the surgical procedure, especially if anterior vitrectomy is also performed. The anchor is usually inserted prior to removal of the lens material. Repositioning and stabilization of the lens capsule significantly facilitates phacoemulsification or aspiration of the lens material and implantation of a posterior chamber IOL.

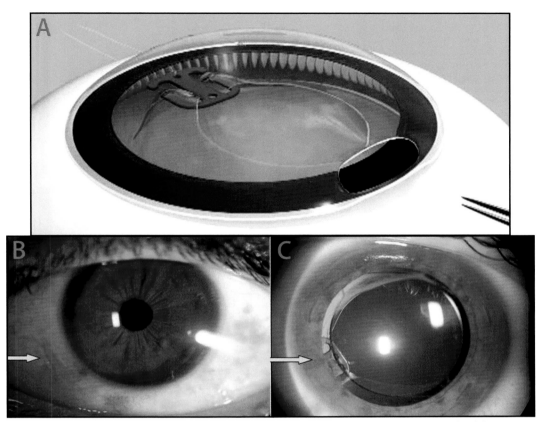

Figure 5-13. Schematic illustration of the capsular AssiAnchor. The 2 lateral arms are located behind the anterior capsule. The anterior central rod is placed in front of the capsule. (Reprinted with permission from Ehud Assia, MD.)

MULTISEGMENTED COLOBOMA RING FOR ANIRIDIA AND MODIFIED CIONNI RING

This multisegmented ring designed by Rasch (Type 50 C; Morcher USA, FCI Ophthalmics, Marshfield Hills, MA) is used in combination with the one of the same kind so that the interspaces of the first ring are covered by the sector shields of the second ring, forming a contiguous artificial iris (Figure 5-14). Dr. Boris Malyugin modified the Cionni ring (Figure 5-15) so that one can load the ring onto the injector and inject the ring.

GLUED ENDOCAPSULAR RING

The glued endocapsular ring device is intended for zonular dialysis greater than 3 clock hours. This concept of transsclerally fixating a portion of the endocapsular ring to achieve greater stability and longevity was shown by Jacob et al[18] and Agarwal and Jacob.[19] For this, the authors designed the glued endocapsular ring which has a haptic that is fixated transsclerally into a Scharioth tunnel. The glued endocapsular ring is manufactured by Epsilon (Irving, TX). This ring is made of a single piece of polyvinylidene fluoride (PVDF) with 3 contiguous parts: a ring

Figure 5-14. Multisegmented Aniridia CTR. Two rings are implanted into the bag. The second ring is then rotated and positioned in such a way that the interspaces of one alternates with the interspaces of the other, thus creating an contiguous artificial iris. (Reprinted with permission from Agarwal A. *Illustrative Guide to Cataract Surgery: A Step-by-Step Approach to Refining Surgical Skills.* Thorofare, NJ: SLACK Incorporated; 2012.)

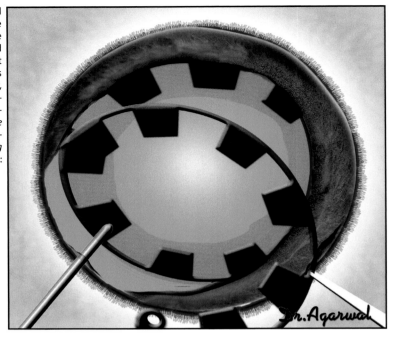

portion, a rhexis-engaging portion, and a haptic (Figure 5-16). The ring portion has 2 arms that are inserted under the rhexis to lie within the capsular fornix. The engaging mechanism has Malyugin ring-like double scrolls,[20] which engage the rim of the rhexis between the 2 scrolls. The haptic is a peripheral extension of the device, which is exteriorized through a 20-gauge sclerotomy made under the scleral flap in the area of dialysis. The excess length is trimmed, and the haptic is tucked into an oblique (coat hanger-shaped) intrascleral Scharioth tunnel[21] made at the edge of the scleral flap with a 26-gauge needle. Once the bag is anchored in position, the surgeon can proceed with phacoemulsification, cortex aspiration, and in-the-bag IOL placement. At the end of surgery, IOL centration is verified and, if required, is adjusted by changing the degree of tuck of the haptic within the tunnel. Vitrectomy is done under the flap, and the flap is glued down over the haptic using fibrin glue. The conjunctiva is also closed with glue (Figure 5-17).

The glued endocapsular ring obviates the need for sutures, providing an inherent stability and longevity that may not be attained with sutured capsular tension segments. Problems associated with sutures such as suture degradation, erosion, knot unraveling, knot exposure, and late IOL subluxation, can be avoided. In addition, the degree of pseudophakodonesis that is seen with sutured fixation is not seen with the glued endocapsular ring. Because the haptics lie within intrascleral tunnels, the glued endocapsular ring is very stable and offers great ease of adjustability. Surgery is easier and more rapid than with suture methods, as complicated intraocular maneuvering with long, thin needles is not required. The fibrin glue seals the flaps hermetically and decreases the chances of postoperative complications, such as wound leak and endophthalmitis.

The glued endocapsular ring is made of the same material (PVDF) and has the same dimension as some IOL haptics. It can be inserted easily into the anterior chamber using the fishtail technique of Angunawela and Little[22] or it can be inserted with arms first and haptics last. With either method, there is no need to tie sutures to the device, which increases the speed and ease of surgery. Because the haptic is exteriorized through a sclerotomy, there is no risk of the glued endocapsular ring falling into the vitreous. Elastic memory allows the ring to regain its shape once it is in the

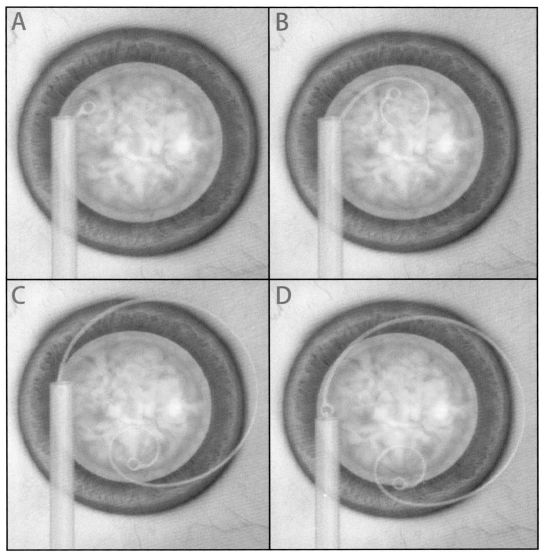

Figure 5-15. Malyugin's modification of the Cionni ring. (A) The tip of the loaded ring is seen protruding through the injector. (B-D) The ring may be injected via the injector into the capsular bag. (Reprinted with permission from Boris Malyugin, MD.)

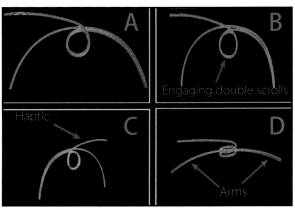

Figure 5-16. The glued endocapsular ring/segment has 2 arms, a double scroll mechanism, and a haptic. It is made of a single-piece of PVDF 130 microns thick. Therefore, is the same material and gauge of an IOL haptic. (A) Glued endocapsular ring. (B) Arrow shows the engaging double scrolls of the device. (C) Arrow shows the haptic of the device. (D) Arrows show the arms of the device.

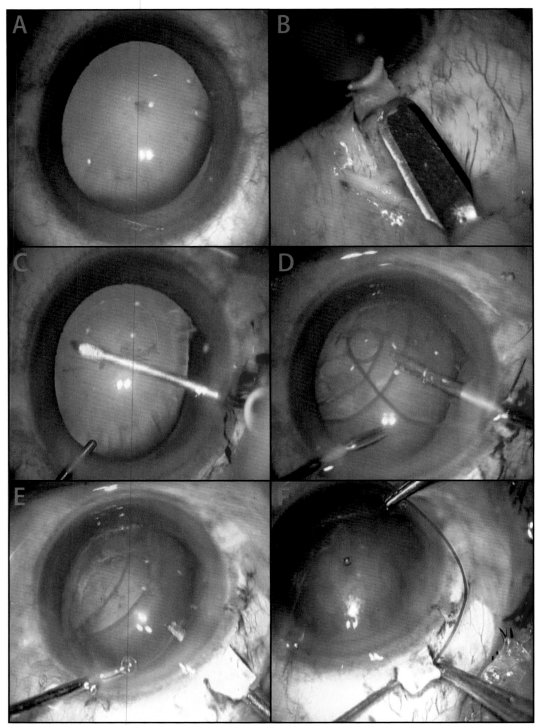

Figure 5-17. Glued endocapsular ring/segment. (A) A subluxated cataract of approximately 180 degrees is shown. (B) A lamellar scleral flap and sclerotomy are created in the area of dialysis. (C) Rhexis is completed. (D) The arms of the device are introduced into the anterior chamber under the rhexis. (E) The haptic is caught by and transferred from hand to hand using 2 end-gripping microforceps—one introduced through the sclerotomy and the other through the sideport until it is caught at the extreme tip by the microforceps introduced through the sclerotomy. (F) The haptic is exteriorized through the sclerotomy.

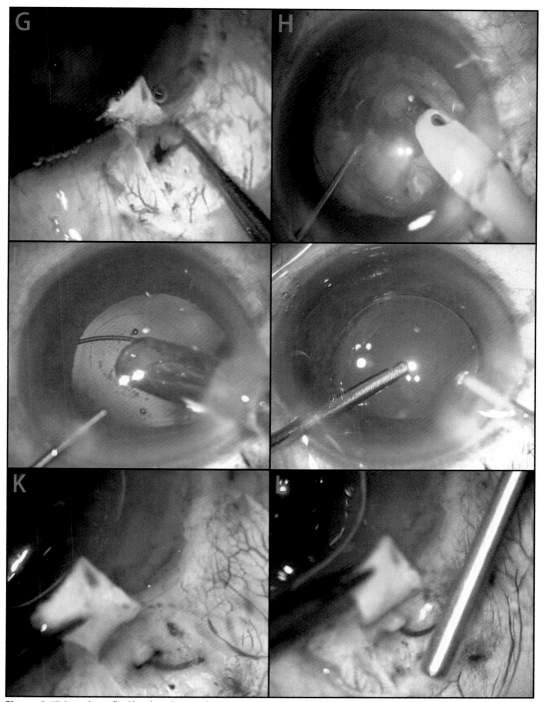

Figure 5-17 (continued). Glued endocapsular ring/segment. (G) The haptic is tucked into an intrascleral Scharioth tunnel. (H) Phacoemulsification is performed. (I) The IOL is implanted. (J) A well-centered IOL is shown. (K) The coathanger type intrascleral tuck hooks the haptic onto the sclera. Further adjustment of IOL centration can be undertaken, if required, by adjusting the degree of tuck of the haptic into the tunnel. (L) Fibrin glue is applied, and the flap is sealed down over the haptic. The conjunctiva is also closed with fibrin glue.

anterior chamber. In the authors' experience with glued IOLs, PVDF has been shown to be inert intrasclerally,[23,24] as was also reported by Scharioth et al.[25] The double scroll engaging mechanism is atraumatic. The device ensures intraoperative and postoperative horizontal and vertical stability of the bag, as well as expansion of the capsular fornix. The robust intraoperative support that the device provides allows safer performance of intracapsular maneuvers, such as in-the-bag nucleus chopping. Explantation, if required, is also relatively simple, which requires the surgeon (under the cover of ophthalmic viscosurgical device) only to grasp the edge of the double scroll and pull the device out through the main port. The flexible device can easily be explanted in this manner.

PATIENT COUNSELING

Because operating on eyes with subluxated cataracts and/or diffuse zonular laxity is more difficult than operating on routine eyes, these patients should be counseled that surgery may not go as hoped and they need to be informed of all the usual risks of cataract surgery. In addition, the patients need to know that surgery will probably take longer. Patients with subluxated cataracts and/or diffuse zonular laxity will not undergo topical anesthesia like so many other patients, and these patients' recovery may be more difficult and prolonged. They may have a fair amount of postoperative astigmatism and require spectacles for correction. They will also experience a greater risk of postoperative retinal detachment. They may experience other postoperative problems including pseudophakodonesis, sunset syndrome, chronic uveitis, cystoid macular edema, and chronic eye pain. These patients should be told they might require suture fixation of the lens implant and that the sutures might not last for the rest of their lives. If the haptics of a posterior chamber lens will be fixated inside scleral pockets, patients should be informed of the possibility that the lens may dislocate if the haptics back their way out of the pockets. If there is a chance patients will be implanted with an anterior chamber model, they should be informed that they will have to exercise care in not rubbing their eye after surgery because doing so may damage the corneal endothelium. These general concerns should be discussed with the patients before surgery. Very specific "after care" instructions should also be discussed, depending on the course of surgery.

FINAL THOUGHTS

Patients with subluxated cataracts and other anomalies of the zonular apparatus generally have significant problems with their vision beyond cataract. Most patients understand the complexity of their situation. Many of these patients have gone from ophthalmologist to ophthalmologist seeking opinions.

It has been the authors' experience that operating on such patients is rewarding. Patients usually experience excellent results and are grateful for the care they received. The authors find this to be the case even when the primary plan was not executed because the intraoperative course did not allow it. Patients are generally forgiving as long as they know that their surgeon planned appropriately and took the steps necessary to assure a good final visual outcome.

Many of these patients come back years later to have their second eye operated, even if it is a completely normal eye. This is a testament to their level of satisfaction with the outcome of surgery on their first eye.

Not every surgeon has the experience to tackle eyes with subluxated cataracts. Such experience develops with time and practice. The beginning surgeon should not feel pressure to keep patients with tough problems inside his or her practice. There is no shame in referring challenging cases to a more experienced surgeon. Challenging cases will usually become easier as the novice surgeon gains more experience.

REFERENCES

1. Hara T, Hara T, Yamada Y. "Equatorial ring" for maintenance of the completely circular contour of the capsular bag equator after cataract removal. *Ophthalmic Surg.* 1991;22;358-359.

2. Hara T, Hara T, Sakanishi K, Yamada Y. Efficacy of equator rings in a experimental rabbit study. *Arch Ophthalmol.* 1995;113:1060-1065.

3. Nagamoto T, Bissen-Miyajima H. A ring to support the capsular bag after continuous curvilinear capsulorrhexis. *J Cataract Refract Surg.* 1994:417-420.

4. Menapace R, Findl O, Georgopoulos M, Rainer G, Vass C, Schmetter K. The capsular tension ring: designs, applications, and techniques. *J Cataract Refract Surg.* 2000;898-912.

5. Nishi O, Hishi K, Sakanishi K, Yamada Y. Explantation of endocapsular posterior chamber lens after spontaneous posterior dislocation. *J Cataract Refract Surg.* 1996,22:272-275.

6. Groessl SA, Anderson CJ. Capsular tension ring in a patient with Weill-Marchesani syndrome. *J Cataract and Refract Surg.* 1998;24:1164-1165.

7. Fischel JD, Wishart MS. Spontaneous complete dislocation of the lens in pseudoexfoliation syndrome. *Eur J Implant Refract Surg.* 1995;7:31-33.

8. Sun R, Gimbel HV. In vitro evaluation of the efficacy of the capsular tension ring for managing zonular dialysis in cataract surgery. *Ophthalmic Surg Lasers.* 1998;29:502-505.

9. Gimble HV, Sun R, Heston JP. Management of zonular dialysis in phacoemulsification and IOL implantation using the capsular tension ring. *Ophthalmic Surg Lasers.* 1997;28:273-281.

10. Gills J, Fenzil R. Intraocular lidocaine causes transient loss of vision in small number of cases. *Ocular Surgery News.* 1996.

11. Agarwal S, Agarwal A, Sachdev MS, Mehta KR, Fine IH, Agarwal A. *Phacoemulsification, Laser Cataract Surgery & Foldable IOLs.* 2nd ed. New Delhi, India: Jaypee Brothers; 2000.

12. Van Cauwenberge F, Rakic JM, Galand A. Complicated posterior capsulorrhexis: etiology, management, and outcome. *Br J Ophthalmol.* 1997;81:195-198.

13. Vass C, Menapace R, Schametter K, et al. Prediction of pseudophakic capsular bag diameter on biometric variables. *J Cataract Refract Surg.* 1999;25:1376-1381.

14. Strenn K, Menapace R, Vass C. Capsular bag shrinkage after implantation of an open loop silicone lens and a polymethyl methacrylate capsule tension ring. *J Cataract Refract Surg.* 1997;23:1543-1547.

15. Nishi O, Nishi K, Menapace R, Akura J. Capsular bending ring to prevent posterior capsule opacification: 2 year follow up. *J Cataract Refract Surg.* 2001;27:1359-1365.

16. Cionni Capsular Tension Rings. Devices for Cataract Surgery—Iris Hooks, Capsular Tension Rings, and More. FCI Ophthalmics. Available at www.fci-ophthalmics.com/cataract#cionni_rings. Accessed June 11, 2013.

17. Kumar DA, Agarwal A. Glued intraocular lens: a major review on surgical technique and results. *Curr Opin Ophthalmol.* 2013;24(1):21-29. doi: 10.1097/ICU.0b013e32835a939f. Review.

18. Jacob S, Agarwal A, Agarwal A, et al. Glued endocapsular hemi-ring segment for fibrin glue-assisted sutureless transscleral fixation of the capsular bag in subluxated cataracts and intraocular lenses. *J Cataract Refract Surg.* 2012;38(2):193-201.

19. Agarwal A, Jacob S. *J Cataract Refract Surg.* Consultation column. February 2013 (in press).

20. Malyugin B. Small pupil phaco surgery: a new technique. *Ann Ophthalmol.* 2007;39:185-193.

21. Gabor SGB, Pavilidis MM. Sutureless intrascleral posterior chamber intraocular lens fixation. *J Cataract Refract Surg.* 2007;33:1851-1854.

22. Angunawela RI, Little B. Fish-tail technique for capsular tension ring insertion. *J Cataract Refract Surg.* 2007;33(5):767-769.

23. Agarwal A, Kumar DA, Jacob S, Baid C, Agarwal A, Srinivasan S. Fibrin glue-assisted sutureless posterior chamber intraocular lens implantation in eyes with deficient posterior capsules. *J Cataract Refract Surg.* 2008;34(9):1433-1438.

24. Kumar DA, Agarwal A. Glued intraocular lens: a major review on surgical technique and results [published online ahead of print October 17, 2012]. *Curr Opin Ophthalmol.*

25. Kumar DA, Agarwal A, Packiyalakshmi S, Jacob S, Agarwal A. Complications and visual outcomes after glued foldable intraocular lens implantation in eyes with inadequate capsules. *J Cataract Refract Surg.* 2013;29. doi: S0886-3350(13)00356-8. 10.1016/j.jcrs.2013.03.004. [Epub ahead of print]

II

Management of Posterior Capsular Rupture

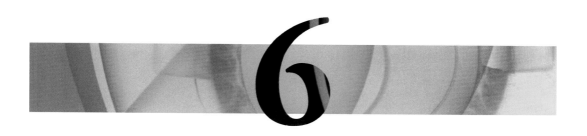

Posterior Capsulorrhexis and Triamcinolone in Posterior Capsular Rupture

Vaishali A. Vasavada, MS and Abhay R. Vasavada, MS, FRCS

A breach in the barrier between the anterior and posterior segments places the eye at an increased risk of posterior segment complications such as retinal detachment, endophthalmitis, and cystoid macular edema.[1-6] Additional intraoperative concerns include early recognition of rupture and vitreous prolapse, carrying out the surgery in a closed chamber, avoiding vitreous prolapse, avoiding high-fluid turbulence and aspiration forces, and coping with nuclear fragments (Figure 6-1).

The broad objectives in the management of a posterior capsular rupture are to prevent vitreous prolapse, perform meticulous removal of the vitreous if it does occur, complete removal of residual lenticular material, and to implant a posterior chamber intraocular lens (IOL), if possible, in the capsular bag. Timely recognition and planned management, depending on the stage of surgery during which the posterior capsular rupture has occurred, is required to ensure an optimal outcome. One should know the role of and strategies for posterior capsulorrhexis in case of posterior capsular rupture and the usefulness of intracameral triamcinolone acetonide in such an event.

ADVANTAGES OF PERFORMING A POSTERIOR CONTINUOUS CURVILINEAR CAPSULORRHEXIS IN CASES OF POSTERIOR CAPSULAR RUPTURE

In a case with a small, relatively central, well-demarcated posterior capsular rupture, converting it into a posterior continuous curvilinear capsulorrhexis (PCCC) provides a continuous and strong margin instead of an irregular, weak margin. A strong continuous margin is important for preventing further extension of the posterior capsular rupture during intraocular maneuvers such as IOL implantation, vitrectomy, and viscoelastic removal. Most importantly, it allows for the

Agarwal A.
*Posterior Capsular Rupture: A Practical Guide
to Prevention and Management* (pp 71-80).
© 2014 Taylor & Francis Group.

Figure 6-1. Posterior capsular rent with nuclear fragment drop. As soon as the surgeon recognizes the posterior capsular rupture, it is important to inject viscoelastic through the sideport before withdrawing the phaco probe. This is because a sudden decompression of the anterior chamber can result in an enlargement of a previously small rent.

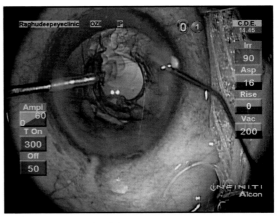

Figure 6-2. In cases with a large rent, the IOL is placed in the sulcus, the optic captured behind the anterior continuous curvilinear capsulorrhexis (ACCC) whenever there is an adequate-sized intact anterior capsule. Avoid placing a single-piece IOL in the sulcus.

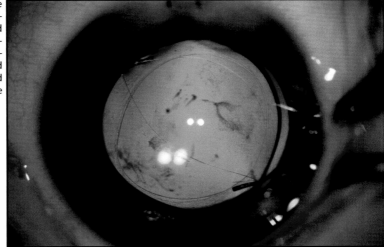

placement of a single-piece, foldable IOL in the capsular bag if the anterior capsulorrhexis is intact (Figure 6-2). In the event that the PCCC is large, a 3-piece IOL can be placed in the ciliary sulcus and captured through the anterior and posterior capsulorhexes.

Converting a posterior capsular rupture into a continuous PCCC is desirable under the following certain situations, which are indications for posterior capsulorrhexis:

- Small size of posterior capsular rupture
- Central or paracentral posterior capsular rupture
- Linear, well-demarcated posterior capsular rupture
- No large radial extensions
- Posterior capsular rupture noticed during last few nuclear fragments removal
- Posterior capsular rupture noticed during irrigation/aspiration (I/A). Once the nuclear fragments and cortex are removed, the posterior capsular rupture can be converted into PCCC.

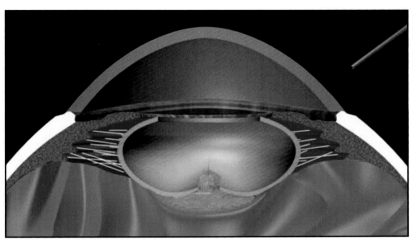

Figure 6-3. Injecting viscoelastic behind the posterior capsular rupture may lead to an extension of the rupture.

TECHNIQUE OF PERFORMING POSTERIOR CONTINUOUS CURVILINEAR CAPSULORRHEXIS

The capsular bag and anterior chamber are filled with high-viscosity sodium hyaluronate prior to initiating PCCC. Care should be taken not to inject excessive viscoelastic behind the open posterior capsule. Gimbel[7] observed that excessive injection through the central puncture may make the posterior capsule convex, which can direct the tear peripherally (Figure 6-3). It is preferable to inject viscoelastic on top of and around the area of the posterior capsular rupture to achieve a flat or concave capsule[8,9] (Figure 6-4).

Microincision capsulorrhexis forceps (Figure 6-5) with a long handle are very useful in performing PCCC as the procedure is initiated by grasping the edge of the posterior capsular rupture with forceps. Thereafter, the PCCC is completed by grasping and regrasping the forceps multiple times. This procedure demands sharp visibility from the operating microscope, as well as a stable eye filled with cohesive viscoelastic. Maintaining high magnification with the operating microscope and dimming the lights in the operating room may aid capsulorrhexis in difficult situations.[10] By frequent grasping and regrasping of the flap (Figure 6-6), it is possible to control the size of the capsulorrhexis and avoid peripheral extension. The forceps should be directed toward the center of the eye and upward toward the corneal endothelium, which helps in preventing peripheral extension of capsulorrhexis. The authors find the use of microincision scissors very useful for converting posterior capsular rupture into PCCC where it is difficult to grasp the flap.

Ideally, the posterior capsulorrhexis should be circular, centric, and smaller than the anterior capsulorrhexis. A desirable size would be 2 to 3 mm. However, it is not always possible to control the size of the PCCC in cases of posterior capsular rupture.

IDENTIFICATION OF AND DEALING WITH VITREOUS PROLAPSE

Anterior vitreous face disruption and vitreous prolapse in the anterior chamber should be carefully looked for in every case. Often, anterior vitreous face disturbance can occur during the maneuver of elevating a flap, or while attempting to regrasp the capsule with the forceps[8,9] (Figure 6-7). Identification and removal of vitreous strands plays a crucial role in ensuring successful outcomes after cataract surgery. Toyofuku et al[11] attributed the risk of retinal detachment to chronic vitreoretinal traction in the anterior vitreous due to cataract removal. Further, prompt

Figure 6-4. Injecting viscoelastic on top of and around the area of the posterior capsular rupture allows the capsular bag to be concave.

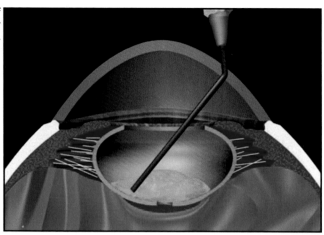

Figure 6-5. Ahmed micrograsper end-opening forceps for PCCC. One can convert posterior capsular rupture to PCCC with microincision capsulorrhexis forceps with a long handle. (Reprinted with permission from MicroSurgical Technology, Redmond, WA.)

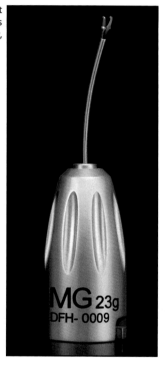

management of prolapsed anterior vitreous by a thorough anterior vitrectomy is the key to preventing further complications.

Surgeons should be vigilant in order to detect signs of anterior vitreous face disturbance. This will help in avoiding further disturbance, thereby optimizing the procedure. However, it may not always be possible to detect small amounts of residual vitreous with the naked eye. Hence, triamcinolone-assisted visualization of the vitreous is recommended because it enhances the detection of residual vitreous strands, thus ensuring a thorough anterior vitrectomy.

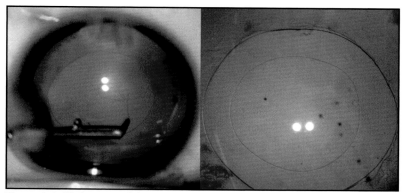

Figure 6-6. (A) Grasping of the posterior capsular flap during PCCC. (B) Posterior capsulorrhexis.

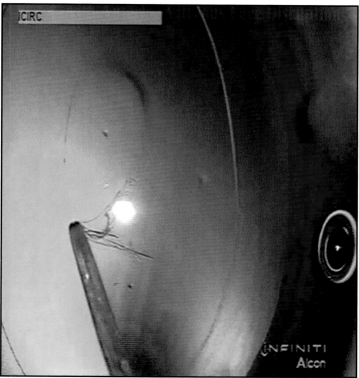

Figure 6-7. Anterior vitreous disturbance, which may be missed during PCCC.

TRIAMCINOLONE ACETONIDE-ASSISTED ANTERIOR VITRECTOMY

Vitreous gel, transparent by design, is virtually invisible under the operating microscope. Vitreoretinal surgeons have been using intravitreal injection of triamcinolone acetonide to visualize the vitreous body during pars plana vitrectomy.[12,13] It has been reported that the granules of triamcinolone acetonide are trapped on the surface of the vitreous body, making it clearly visible

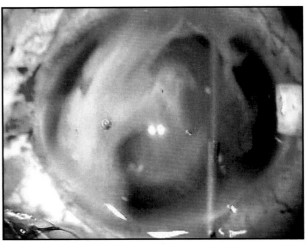

under the surgical microscope. Further, the intracameral use of triamcinolone (Figure 6-8) has also been reported to visualize the presence of vitreous in the anterior chamber after posterior capsular rupture in adults.[15,16] Several published reports have described strategies for visualizing vitreous disturbance during adult cataract surgery using triamcinolone acetonide.[14,15]

In the presence of anterior vitreous face disturbance, these particles tend to become entrapped and impregnated in the vitreous gel, clearly defining the extent of vitreous disturbance and its presence in the anterior chamber (Figure 6-9). On the other hand, an intact vitreous face appears as a convex, bulging structure (Figure 6-10). Further, with an intact vitreous face, triamcinolone acetonide tends to swirl freely when injected within the rhexis margin.

Previously, a few authors[14,15] have used preservative-containing triamcinolone acetonide in a dose of 4 mg/mL to identify vitreous prolapse in cases of posterior capsular rupture. These authors have used microfilters to remove the preservative. The authors previously described the use of preservative-free triamcinolone acetonide (Aurocort) in the same dosage as recommended but without any microfilters, as this preparation does not contain preservative.[16] Therefore, this drug is safe to use in the anterior chamber, and needs no further processing. Several studies have shown that it is not the triamcinolone itself but the preservative (benzyl alcohol) that is responsible for its toxic effect.[17,18] This suspension is injected directly (filtration procedures are not needed), thus minimizing possible errors associated with filtration procedures. Preservative-free triamcinolone acetonide is injected intracamerally to help with visualization, thereby more effectively removing any residual vitreous strands in the anterior chamber.

CREATING A SUSPENSION

Aurocort comes in a vial with a concentration of 40 mg/mL. From this vial, 0.5 mL of the drug is withdrawn in a 5-mL syringe containing 4.5 mL of balanced salt solution (BSS) to achieve the desired concentration of 4 mg/mL. Next, 1 mL of this Aurocort suspension is withdrawn into a tuberculin syringe, and a total of 0.2 mL is injected thrice during the surgery. Extreme care should be taken to avoid the triamcinolone acetonide from clumping by shaking it thoroughly to ensure a uniform suspension before withdrawing the drug into the syringe. After withdrawal, the suspension should be injected immediately into the anterior chamber to prevent precipitation of the triamcinolone particles in the syringe.

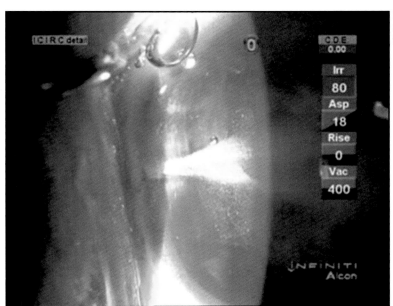

Figure 6-9. Vitreous strands made visible by staining with triamcinolone acetonide.

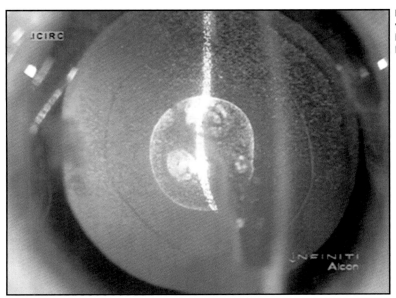

Figure 6-10. Intact anterior vitreous face, seen as a convex, bulging structure highlighted by triamcinolone acetonide.

INJECTING PRESERVATIVE-FREE TRIAMCINOLONE ACETONIDE

Triamcinolone acetonide is injected 3 times during the surgery.

- First injection: 0.1 mL triamcinolone acetonide is injected into the anterior chamber once the posterior capsular rupture is recognized. Any vitreous prolapse will be identified as white strands in the anterior chamber. In the absence of vitreous prolapse, the triamcinolone acetonide will be seen to swirl freely in the anterior chamber. Adequate bimanual anterior vitrectomy is performed to remove vitreous in the anterior chamber.

- Second injection: After performing the initial vitrectomy and PCCC, a second injection of 0.1 mL triamcinolone acetonide is given. This will help to identify any residual vitreous strands in the anterior chamber.

- Third injection: 0.1 mL of triamcinolone acetonide is injected following IOL implantation to detect the presence of vitreous. Thereafter, I/A is performed to remove the triamcinolone as well as ophthalmic viscosurgical device (OVD). In the event vitreous strands are seen, a vitrectomy is performed again.

Triamcinolone is then rinsed off with BSS and all the incisions are sutured with 10-0 nylon. Finally, 0.1 mL of 0.5% moxifloxacin (Vigamox) can be injected into the anterior chamber at the end of surgery. It is important to suture these incisions to avoid any leaks or chamber shallowing postoperatively.

CONCERNS WITH THE USE OF PRESERVATIVE CONTAINING TRIAMCINOLONE ACETONIDE

Concern has been raised regarding the toxicity of commercially available triamcinolone on corneal endothelium, retinal pigment epithelial cells, and lens epithelial cells.[17,18] Dada et al[19] reported the use of the Aurocort administered via the pars plana route, and have found it to be safe and effective. Some surgeons might argue that clinical signs suggestive of vitreous strands may be sufficient in detecting residual vitreous strands. However, we believe that, at times, it is difficult to visualize the vitreous strands due to the transparent nature of the vitreous and retroillumination of the microscope.

In the literature, major concerns with the use of triamcinolone acetonide in adults include the occurrence of glaucoma[14,15] and sterile endophthalmitis.[20-24] Increased intraocular pressure (IOP) is known to occur with the intraocular use of triamcinolone acetonide. In one clinical study,[5] only one eye had an increase in IOP, and the authors suggested that triamcinolone acetonide granules plug up the trabecular meshwork and inhibit aqueous outflow. Because there was no apparent increase in IOP in the other eyes, the authors suggested that intracameral triamcinolone might not necessarily induce an increase in IOP when triamcinolone acetonide granules are removed. In another study,[23] the authors reported in pediatric eyes that intracameral diagnostic use of preservative-free triamcinolone acetonide did not lead to increased IOP.

It is important to remember that triamcinolone can sometimes stain the viscoelastic in the anterior chamber. However, there are a few differences in the staining pattern. Generally, viscoelastic forms a diffuse uniform pattern of staining and is aspirated very quickly in a bolus, whereas with vitreous disturbance, the staining pattern is localized to the vitreous strands. This needs to be kept in mind when the surgeon uses triamcinolone in the anterior chamber in a viscoelastic-filled eye.

INTRAOCULAR LENS IMPLANTATION IN THE CAPSULAR BAG IN CASES OF POSTERIOR CAPSULAR RUPTURE

Converting a posterior capsular rupture into a PCCC ensures in-the-bag IOL implantation without the risk of extending the posterior capsular rupture. An adequate vitrectomy should be performed if there is vitreous prolapse, following which IOL implantation is performed. A single-piece, foldable IOL may be implanted in the bag. In a case with posterior capsular rupture, if the incision is tight and small, it should be enlarged so that the IOL can be injected without further distortion of the eye. The material and design of the IOL selected should be such that there is slow and controlled unfolding of the IOL in the capsular bag.

CONCLUSION

If the posterior capsular rupture is localized, converting it into a PCCC ensures a strong, stable capsulorrhexis margin, which prevents further extension of the posterior capsular rupture and allows in-the-bag placement of the IOL. The use of microcapsulorrhexis forceps allows maintenance of a closed chamber during PCCC. A high-viscosity cohesive viscoelastic should be used. Frequent grasping and regrasping of the posterior capsular flap will allow a continuous, controlled PCCC. Vitreous management is the key in deciding the postoperative fate of the eye with a posterior capsular rupture. The role of preservative-free triamcinolone acetonide in making vitreous visible to the surgeon cannot be overemphasized. Preservative-free triamcinolone acetonide should be kept ready in the operating room.

REFERENCES

1.   Javitt JC, Vitale S, Canner JK, et al. National outcomes of cataract extraction. Endophthalmitis following inpatient surgery. *Arch Ophthalmol.* 1991;109(8):1085-1089.
2.   Kraff MC, Sanders DR, Jampol LM, Lieberman HL. Effect of primary capsulotomy with extracapsular surgery on incidence of pseudophakic cystoid macular edema. *Am J Ophthalmol.* 1984;98:166-170.
3.   Gonvers M. New approach to managing vitreous loss and dislocated lens fragments during phacoemulsification. *J Cataract Refract Surg.* 1994;20:346-349.
4.   Nprregard JC, Thoning H, Nernth-Petersen P, et al. Risk of endophthalmitis after cataract extraction: results from the international cataract surgery outcomes study. *Br J Ophthalmol.* 1997;81:102-106.
5.   Powell SK, Olsen RJ. Incidence of retinal detachment after cataract surgery and neodymium:YAG laser capsulotomy. *J Cataract Refract Surg.* 1995;21:132-135.
6.   Yoshida A, Ogasawaha H, Jalkh AE, et al. Retinal detachment after cataract surgery: predisposing factors. *Ophthalmology.* 1992;99:453-459.
7.   Gimbel HV, Sun R, Ferensowics M, et al. Intraoperative management of posterior capsule tears in phacoemulsification and intraocular lens implantation. *Ophthalmology.* 2001;108(12):2186-2189.
8.   Dholakia SA, Praveen MR, Vasavada AR, et al. Completion rate of primary posterior continuous curvilinear capsulorrhexis and vitreous disturbance during congenital cataract surgery. *J AAPOS.* 2006;10:351-356.
9.   Praveen MR, Vasavada AR, Koul A, Trivedi RH, et al. Subtle signs of anterior vitreous face disturbance during posterior capsulorrhexis in pediatric cataract surgery. *J Cataract Refract Surg.* 2008;34:163-167.
10.   Haussman N, Richard G. Investigations on diathermy for anterior capsulotomy. *Invest Ophthalmol Vis Sci.* 1991;32:2155-2159.
11.   Toyofuku H, Hirose T, Schepens CL. Retinal detachment following congenital cataract surgery. Preoperative findings in 114 eyes. *Arch Ophthalmol.* 1980;98(4):669-675.
12.   Peyman GA, Cheema R, Conway MD, et al. Triamcinolone acetonide as an aid to visualization of the vitreous and the posterior hyaloid during pars plana vitrectomy. *Retina.* 2000;20(5):554-555.
13.   Tano Y, Chandler D, Machemer R. Treatment of intraocular proliferation with intravitreal injection of triamcinolone acetonide. *Am J Ophthalmol.* 1980;90(6):810-816.
14.   Burk SE, Da Mata AP, Snyder ME, et al. Visualizing vitreous using Kenalog suspension. *J Cataract Refract Surg.* 2003;29(4):645-651.
15.   Yamakiri K, Uchino E, Kimura K, et al. Intracameral triamcinolone helps to visualize and remove the vitreous body in anterior chamber in cataract surgery. *Am J Ophthalmol.* 2004;138(4):650-652.
16.   Shah SK, Vasavada V, Praveen MR, Vasavada AR, Trivedi RH, Dixit NV. Triamcinolone-assisted vitrectomy in pediatric cataract surgery. *J Cataract Refract Surg.* 2009;35:230-232.
17.   Chang YS, Wu CL, Tseng SH, Kuo PY, Tseng SY. Cytotoxicity of triamcinolone acetonide on human retinal pigment epithelial cells. *Invest Ophthalmol Vis Sci.* 2007;48(6):2792-2798.
18.   Maia M, Farah ME, Belfort RN, et al. Effects of intravitreal triamcinolone acetonide injection with and without preservative. *Br J Ophthalmol.* 2007;91(9):1122-1124.
19.   Dada T, Dhawan M, Garg S, et al. Safety and efficacy of intraoperative intravitreal injection of triamcinolone acetonide injection after phacoemulsification in cases of uveitic cataract. *J Cataract Refract Surg.* 2007;33(9):1613-1618.
20.   Jonas JB, Kreissig I, Degenring RF. Endophthalmitis after intravitreal injection of triamcinolone. *Arch Ophthalmol.* 2003;121:1663-1664.

21. Nelson ML, Tennant MTS, Sivalingam A, et al. Infectious and presumed noninfectious endophthalmitis after intravitreal triamcinolone acetonide injection. *Retina.* 2003;23:686-691.

22. Moshfeghi DM, Kaiser PK, Scott IU, et al. Acute endophthalmitis following intravitreal triamcinolone acetonide injection. *Am J Ophthalmol.* 2003;136:791-796.

23. Sakamoto T, Enaida H, Kubota T, et al. Incidence of acute endophthalmitis after triamcinolone-assisted pars plana vitrectomy. *Am J Ophthalmol.* 2004;38:137-138.

24. Praveen MR, Shah SK, Vasavada VA, et al. Triamcinolone-assisted vitrectomy in pediatric cataract surgery: intraoperative effectiveness and postoperative outcome. *J AAPOS.* 2010;14:340-344.

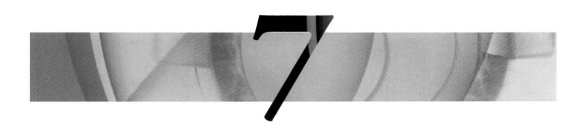

Technique of Anterior Vitrectomy for the Cataract Surgeon

Som Prasad, MS, FRCSEd, FACS, FRCOphth

D ue to improving techniques, the incidence of posterior capsular tear seems to have decreased over the years,[1] but it still remains in the region of 2% in most large series studies reported recently.[1,2] Less frequently, nuclear fragments may be displaced into the vitreous cavity.[3] These uncommon occurrences place the cataract surgeon in a less than comfortable zone because the operating room staff and the surgeon may not be as well prepared as they would like to be.[4] It is essential for the cataract surgeon to become familiar with the vitrectomy machine being used and know the technique for performing anterior vitrectomy. Anterior vitrectomy may be performed via a wound that is anterior to the iris plane or behind the iris plane (ie, pars plana vitrectomy). Both approaches have associated risks and benefits. Familiarity with one or both vitrectomy techniques and preparing the surgical team will be beneficial for the cataract surgeon. Once the situation has been stabilized, bimanual anterior vitrectomy is the standard approach that should be used.

VITRECTOMY PROBE

The surgeon must familiarize him- or herself with the available instrumentation, especially when moving to a new operating room setting. Full-function vitrectomy probes with an irrigating sleeve over the cutter should be avoided. It is more useful to use a separate irrigation line placed through a sideport incision and an active instrument placed through a separate incision to remove the vitreous.

SIGNS OF CAPSULAR TEAR

The classic signs of capsular tear are a sudden deepening of the anterior chamber and pupil dilation, also known as the *pupil snap sign*, occurring due to abrupt equalization of hydrostatic

Agarwal A.
Posterior Capsular Rupture: A Practical Guide
to Prevention and Management (pp 81-86).
© 2014 Taylor & Francis Group.

Figure 7-1. Triamcinolone helps to identify presenting vitreous after vitreous loss to guide anterior vitrectomy.

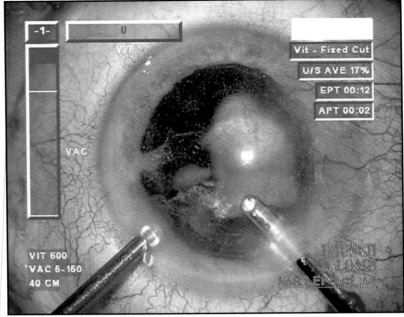

pressure between the anterior and posterior segments. However, vitreous loss can occur with more subtle signs, such as when the nucleus moves less readily than expected or when vitreous blocks the phaco tip. Generally, if the surgeon suspects that a capsule tear has occurred, it probably has, and the surgical strategy must be changed.

IMMEDIATE MANAGEMENT

Phacoemulsification and aspiration should be immediately stopped. Irrigation is continued to keep the anterior chamber stable. The phaco probe is kept stable, the second instrument is removed, and viscoelastic is injected through the sideport. As the anterior chamber is stabilized, the bottle height is lowered (from 20 to 40 cm), and irrigation is eased off. The phaco probe is withdrawn without collapsing the anterior chamber.

BIMANUAL ANTERIOR VITRECTOMY

At this stage, assess the remaining nuclear segments, the site, the extent of the capsular tear, and presenting vitreous. If small nuclear fragments remain, move them away from the site of the tear with an ophthalmic viscosurgical device (OVD) and guide them out of the wound, which may be extended to facilitate removal. Any nuclear segments moving posteriorly should never be chased. It is safer to manage the anterior segment and leave any posteriorly dislocated nuclear fragments for a vitreoretinal specialist to manage. It is useful to inject a small amount of triamcinolone acetonide (Kenalog), used off-label, into the anterior chamber at this stage. The triamcinolone crystals adhere to any vitreous that has presented, greatly facilitating visualization (Figure 7-1).

A second sideport incision is then created. Surgeons should not use the cutter through the phaco incision because it can cause anterior chamber shallowing, as the width of the instrument is usually smaller than the incision used for phacoemulsification. If unstable, the main incision should be secured with a suture. The infusion cannula is placed through a sideport with a low bottle height and the fluid flow is directed toward the anterior chamber angle. The cutter goes through the second sideport, establishing a stable, closed system. A high cut rate and low flow are advisable; the cutting rate should be set at the highest rate allowable on the phaco machine, which ranges from 600 to 5,000 cpm on various models, and vacuum set at 150 to 200 mm Hg. This minimizes the risk of retinal traction while the vitreous is cut and removed.

The cutter is placed through the tear with the cutting port positioned behind the posterior capsule. Most of the anterior vitreous is drawn backward and efficiently removed. The cutter is then moved forward into the capsular bag to deal with any remaining lens matter, with the cut rate set at 300 cpm and increased vacuum to draw the firmer lens material into the cutting port. The cortex is removed next, using the vacuum-only setting of the cutter. The cortex is freed and drawn into the center, and the cutting action is activated to remove it. The cutter is withdrawn, and OVD fills the anterior chamber.

INTRAOCULAR LENS IMPLANTATION

In most cases, there is adequate capsular support to implant an intraocular lens (IOL) into the ciliary sulcus. The overall diameter of the chosen IOL should be at least 13 mm. If there is a small central tear that can be converted into a posterior capsulorrhexis, then in-the-bag implantation is often safe. Alternatively, if the capsulorrhexis is intact, optic capture can be used to place a lens with the optics behind the anterior capsule and the haptics in the sulcus. In cases where there is no capsule, one can use the glued IOL technique.

OVD is removed from the anterior chamber with no attempt being made to remove it from behind the IOL. The pupil is then constricted with an agent such as acetylcholine chloride (Miochol-E). It is often useful to place a small amount of triamcinolone in the anterior chamber again at this point to identify any errant strands of vitreous. The triamcinolone is then flushed with irrigation/aspiration (I/A). If wound integrity is in any doubt, put in a suture.

DRY ANTERIOR VITRECTOMY

An alternative approach is to use a dry technique, in which vitreous is cut and removed without an infusion. This is especially useful for small amounts of vitreous presenting toward the end of a procedure (eg, if a strand of vitreous presents through a small area of zonular loss toward the end of cortical clean-up or after IOL implantation). In this setting, it is efficient to refill the anterior chamber with viscoelastic and cut and remove the strand of vitreous with the cutter (Figure 7-2). As minimal maneuvering is required—and only a small volume is removed—the anterior chamber will not collapse and the surgical goal is rapidly achieved. A dispersive viscoelastic will tamponade the vitreous and is preferred in this setting. A useful tip to prevent chamber collapse when performing a dry anterior vitrectomy is to have a syringe of viscoelastic in the nondominant hand through the sideport and use this to top off the viscoelastic fill as the vitrectomy proceeds.

PARS PLANA APPROACH

Increasingly, using a single pars plana entry has been advocated for anterior vitrectomy. Although conceptually enticing, this approach requires a separate skill set that may not be available to all anterior segment surgeons.[5] The attraction of the pars plana approach is that vitreous moves in an anterior to posterior direction (as opposed to the anterior approach used in bimanual

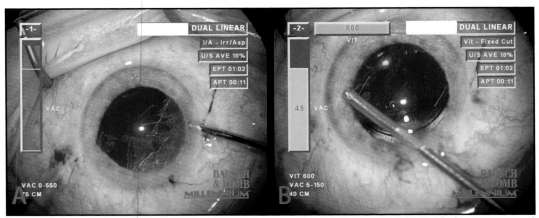

Figure 7-2. Dry anterior vitrectomy. (A) Vitreous strand presents through the zonule at the 9 o'clock position toward the end of cortical clean-up. This is tamponaded by viscoelastic and most of the cortex is removed without disturbing this limited amount of presenting vitreous. (B) After IOL implantation in the bag, the cutter is used to remove the vitreous strand in a viscoelastic-filled anterior chamber without infusion.

anterior vitrectomy when vitreous is drawn forward) to be removed. One also achieves enhanced and more controlled access to the rest of the lens matter. Cortical material, epinucleus, and even nuclear material that is not very hard may be removed by the Ocutome (Bausch + Lomb, Rochester, NY) by lowering the cut rate and increasing vacuum slightly.

There are also certain situations where the only practical approach is to use a pars plana incision to remove vitreous, enabling cataract surgery to proceed. A crowded eye with a shallow anterior chamber,[6] or even an eye with a nonexistent anterior chamber due to phacomorphic glaucoma[7] or aqueous misdirection are best managed by using a pars plana incision to remove some vitreous, thus allowing for reformation of the anterior chamber. Therefore, the pars plana approach should be an essential skill in the repertoire of the anterior segment surgeon.

To briefly explain, the pars plana technique uses an infusion through the sideport and makes a single pars plana incision 3.5 mm behind the limbus (Figure 7-3). The cutter is then placed into the vitreous cavity. This can be done after reflecting the conjunctiva with a MVR blade for a 20-gauge cutter or transconjunctivally using a 25-gauge trocar cannula system for a high-speed, 25-gauge cutter. This allows the flow to move in one direction—from anterior to posterior—making removal of vitreous more efficient. Many anterior segment surgeons may not be familiar or comfortable with pars plana incisions; therefore, the author highlights the nuances and surgical pearls that will allow the deployment of this technique in a safe and predictable manner.

As with any surgical technique, it is essential to learn the steps of the procedure. The first principle is to maintain a closed chamber at all times. Hypotony must be avoided throughout. If there is any doubt about the competency of the corneal incision, it should be closed with a temporary suture prior to the pars plana incision being made. This avoids hypotony and also facilitates the pars plana incision, which requires a firm eye. If performing surgery under topical anesthesia, remember that the pars plana incision will be uncomfortable; therefore, it is advisable to administer a small amount of subconjunctival anesthetic in the area of the planned incision. The importance of constantly explaining the situation to the patient, sometimes termed "vocal anesthesia" cannot be overemphasized. With a firm eye and adequate anesthesia, one can either use an MVR blade after taking the conjunctiva down or a transconjunctival approach. Incisions should always be bevelled to allow for better sealing at the end of the procedure (Figure 7-4). The highest cut rate possible should be used to reduce retinal traction. Remember, even in an eye with a complete posterior vitreous detachment, the vitreous remains attached to the vitreous base, which is the region in which most retinal tears occur in pseudophakic eyes. A high cut rate with

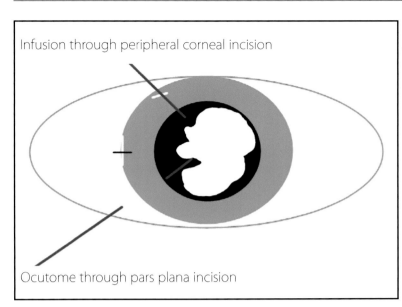

Infusion through peripheral corneal incision

Ocutome through pars plana incision

Figure 7-3. Schematic diagram showing infusion through a peripheral corneal incision and vitrectomy probe placed though a pars plana incision. A temporary suture closes the phaco incision to avoid leakage and hypotony.

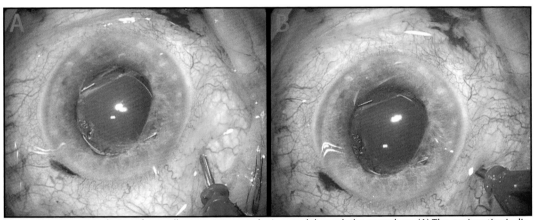

Figure 7-4. Correct technique for small-gauge trocars to be inserted through the pars plana. (A) The conjunctiva is displaced and the trocar enters the pars plana 3.5 mm behind the limbus, initially at an acute angle. (B) Once the cannula has engaged the sclera, the direction of the approach is changed to a perpendicular direction. This results in a 2-plane bevelled incision in the sclera that self-seals when the cannula is removed at the end of the procedure.

low to moderate vacuum reduces this risk. Therefore, although it may be counterintuitive to put the "foot to metal," that is what needs to be done. Once vitreous has been removed, the cut rate can be lowered to remove any remaining lens matter. Small-gauge transconjunctival incisions self-seal when the port is removed, but it is necessary to suture a 20-gauge scleral incision and to also close the conjunctiva over it.

POSTOPERATIVE CARE

It is important to manage postoperative inflammation and intraocular pressure (IOP) well. Finally, detailed fundus and full peripheral examinations must be obtained. It is very important to visualize and check the peripheral retina before the patient is discharged, as the risk of retinal tears is increased whenever a posterior capsular tear occurs, and there is the risk of entry site tears with any pars plana incisions. It is also important to clearly explain to the patient the warning signs of retinal tears and encourage the patient to seek urgent medical attention in the unlikely event that they should happen.

CONCLUSION

Effective management, with good surgical technique and postoperative care, will, in most cases, ensure excellent visual outcomes, even when vitreous loss occurs during cataract surgery.

REFERENCES

1. Lundström M, Behndig A, Kugelberg M, Montan P, Stenevi U, Thorburn W. Decreasing rate of capsule complications in cataract surgery: eight-year study of incidence, risk factors, and data validity by the Swedish National Cataract Register. *J Cataract Refract Surg.* 2011;37(10):1762-1767.
2. Narendran N, Jaycock P, Johnston RL, et al. The Cataract National Dataset electronic multicentre audit of 55,567 operations: risk stratification for posterior capsule rupture and vitreous loss. *Eye (Lond).* 2009;23(1):31-37.
3. Mahmood S, von Lany H, Cole MD, et al. Displacement of nuclear fragments into the vitreous complicating phacoemulsification surgery in the UK: incidence and risk factors. *Br J Ophthalmol.* 2008;92(4):488-492.
4. Arbisser LB. Managing intraoperative complications in cataract surgery. *Curr Opin Ophthalmol.* 2004;15(1):33-39.
5. Chalam KV, Gupta SK, Vinjamaram S, Shah VA. Small-gauge, sutureless pars plana vitrectomy to manage vitreous loss during phacoemulsification. *J Cataract Refract Surg.* 2003;29(8):1482-1486.
6. MacKool RJ. Pars plana vitreous tap for phacoemulsification in the crowded eye. *J Cataract Refract Surg.* 2002;28(4):572-573.
7. Dada T, Kumar S, Gadia R, et al. Sutureless single-port transconjunctival pars plana limited vitrectomy combined with phacoemulsification for management of phacomorphic glaucoma. *J Cataract Refract Surg.* 2007;33(6):951-954.

8

Intraocular Lens Scaffold and Glued Intraocular Lens Scaffold Techniques

Athiya Agarwal, MD, DO and Amar Agarwal, MS, FRCS, FRCOphth

Posterior capsular rupture[1-3] with vitreous prolapse and the nucleus still in the capsular bag is an impending situation for a nucleus drop. As a preventive step, it is usual for the cataract surgeon to extend the corneal incision and deliver the nucleus.[4-6] Lens glide or ophthalmic viscosurgical device-assisted (eg, sodium chondroitin sulfate/sodium hyaluronate ophthalmic [Viscoat]) levitation has also been used to remove nuclear fragments.[7,8] Another method is to emulsify the nucleus in the anterior chamber with low flow rate and vacuum. Although a small fragment, which descends into the vitreous, may be left for observation, larger nuclear fragments always require surgical removal.[9,10] Nucleus drop can induce vitritis and macular edema, thereby affecting best-corrected vision.[10] A second surgery for retrieving the dropped nucleus can cause additional trauma to the eye.

INTRAOCULAR LENS SCAFFOLD

The intraocular lens (IOL) scaffold technique[11,12] refers to a foldable IOL being used as a scaffold to prevent the nucleus fragments from descending into the vitreous in cases of posterior capsular rupture. After removing the vitreous in the anterior chamber by anterior vitrectomy, the nuclear fragments are levitated into the anterior chamber and supported on the iris. A 3-piece, foldable IOL is injected via the existing corneal incision with one haptic above the iris and the other haptic extending outside the incision. Alternatively, both haptics can be placed above the iris or above the capsule. The nucleus is emulsified with the phaco probe above the IOL optic. Cortical cleaning is done and the IOL is then placed over the remnants of the capsule in the ciliary sulcus. This procedure can be performed in eyes with moderate to soft cataracts because it avoids corneal incision extension and thereby limits induced astigmatism. This technique was conceptualized by Dr. Amar Agarwal.

Agarwal A.
Posterior Capsular Rupture: A Practical Guide to Prevention and Management (pp 87-97).
© 2014 Taylor & Francis Group.

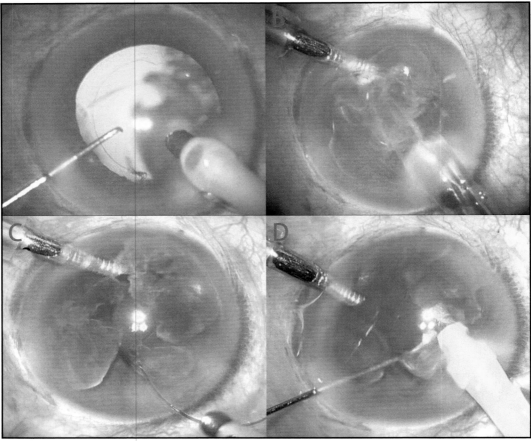

Figure 8-1. IOL scaffold technique. (A) Posterior capsular rupture during epinucleus removal. (B) Anterior chamber maintainer is placed. Foldable IOL is injected through the clear corneal wound. (C) One haptic is placed over the iris and the other is placed outside of the incision. (D) Epinucleus is removed with a phaco probe.

The word *scaffold* comes from the medieval Latin word *scaffaldus*, meaning a temporary platform. In the IOL scaffold technique, the 3-piece IOL acts as a temporary platform and prevents the nuclear fragments from falling into the vitreous cavity.

SURGICAL TECHNIQUE

When there is a posterior capsular rupture with retained nuclear fragments (Figure 8-1A), an anterior chamber maintainer is introduced through a 1.2-mm stab microvitreoretinal (MVR) blade incision (Figure 8-1B). The position of the anterior chamber maintainer should be away from the posterior capsular rupture, and flow should be kept low. Anterior vitrectomy is performed with the vitrectomy cutter to remove the vitreous prolapsed in the anterior chamber. An Agarwal globe stabilization rod (Katena Products, Denville, NJ), which is passed through the sideport, helps to push the fragment away from the posterior capsular rupture. The fragments are brought into the anterior chamber to rest on the iris. A foldable IOL is then injected via the existing corneal wound and is maneuvered below the nucleus (see Figure 8-1B). The leading haptic of the IOL is positioned above the iris, and the trailing haptic is placed just outside the incision site (Figure 8-1C). Using a dialer in the nondominant hand, the junction of the optic haptic junction on the trailing side

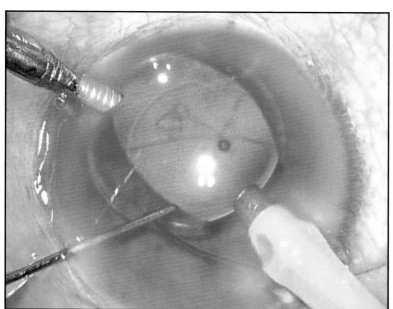

Figure 8-2. The nondominant hand adjusts the optic-haptic junction so that the IOL is well-centered while emulsifying the epinucleus.

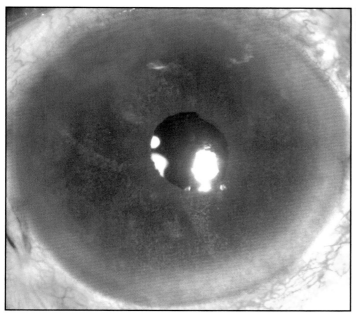

Figure 8-3. Clinical photograph of the patient 1 month after an IOL scaffold procedure.

is maneuvered so that the IOL blocks the pupil. Thus, the IOL acts as a scaffold and prevents the fragments from falling into the vitreous cavity (Figure 8-1D). The nuclear fragment is then removed with the phaco probe (low flow and vacuum; see Figure 8-1D). Cortex is removed by alternating between vitrector and aspiration modes using a vitrectomy probe with suction and low aspiration. The nondominant hand adjusts the trailing optic haptic junction so that the IOL is well-centered over the pupil, acting as a scaffold while emulsifying the nucleus (Figure 8-2). Once cortical clean-up is done, the IOL is placed over the capsular remnants in the ciliary sulcus. The anterior chamber maintainer is then removed and wound hydration is carried out. Postoperatively, topical antibiotic and corticosteroid eye drops are used 4 times daily for 2 weeks (Figure 8-3). A

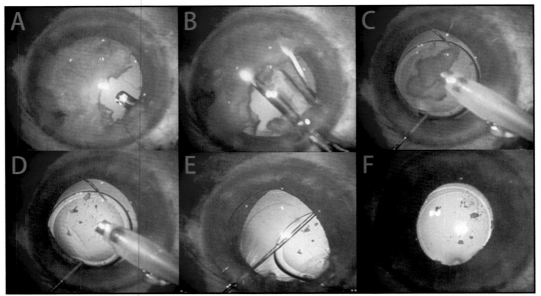

Figure 8-4. IOL scaffold technique with 23-gauge trocar infusion and moderately soft nucleus. (A) Posterior capsular rupture during nucleus removal. (B) Foldable IOL is injected through the clear corneal wound. (C) Nucleus removed with phaco probe above the IOL optic. (D) Cortical aspiration done. (E) IOL pushed into the ciliary sulcus. (F) IOL well-centered at the end of surgery. (Reprinted with permission from Kumar DA, Agarwal A, Prakash G, et al. IOL scaffold technique for posterior capsular rupture. *J Refract Surg.* 2012;28(5):314-315.)

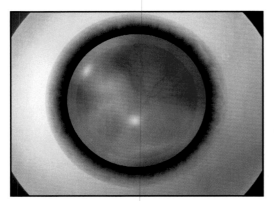

Figure 8-5. Posterior capsular rupture.

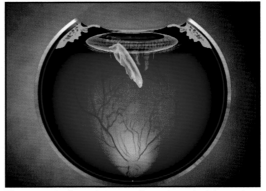

Figure 8-6. Posterior capsular rupture with nucleus sinking.

short-acting mydriatic drop twice a day is used for the initial 3 days postoperatively. Instead of an anterior chamber maintainer, one can also use a sutureless trocar cannula system.

This technique can be easily done in moderately soft nuclei (Figure 8-4). In hard cataracts with posterior capsular rupture occurring before disassembly of nucleus, it might be better to extend the incision and remove the nucleus in total to avoid corneal damage.

ADVANTAGES

Although other techniques can be performed to prevent nucleus fragments from descending into the vitreous after intraoperative posterior capsular rupture, this method of using the IOL as a scaffold has not been reported earlier[11] (Figures 8-5 to 8-8). Conversion of phacoemulsification

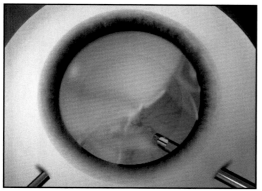

Figure 8-7. Vitrectomy.

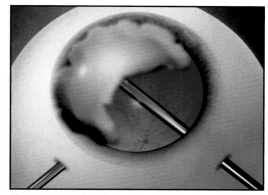

Figure 8-8. Nucleus brought anteriorly above the iris.

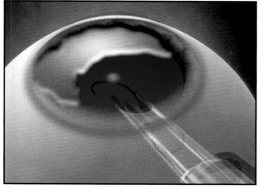

Figure 8-9. Three-piece IOL is injected into the anterior chamber.

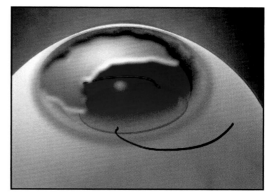

Figure 8-10. Three-piece IOL is positioned with one haptic above the iris and the other haptic outside of the corneal incision.

to extracapsular cataract extraction (ECCE)[4,5] is done when a large nucleus still remains. Some surgeons prefer to use the Sheets' glide (Beaver-Visitec International, MA) to deliver the nucleus. Corneal wound extension is required in both methods, which can increase the risk of postoperative complications such as suture-induced astigmatism, postoperative wound leak, shallow anterior chamber, and endophthalmitis. Another technique for nucleus removal is the phaco sandwich method,[6] where a vectis and spatula are used. However, the incision in a phaco sandwich is sclerocorneal and requires extension. Viscoat-assisted posterior levitation[7] is performed in eyes with nucleus displaced into the anterior vitreous, followed by nucleus emulsification with a phaco probe above a trimmed Sheets' glide[8] after wound extension. The Sheets' glide requires the incision to be extended.

Another technique for preventing fragment drop during phacoemulsification in PCR is Dr. Keiki Mehta's hydroxyethyl methacrylate (HEMA) life boat.[13] For this, a contact lens is injected between the iris and the nucleus to prevent the nucleus from falling down. The contact lens is removed after nucleus emulsification. Unlike the IOL scaffold, this technique requires explantation of an implanted device. In the IOL scaffold technique, the corneal wound remains intact and there is no wound extension and no need for suturing, thus decreasing the chances for induced astigmatism (Figures 8-9 to 8-14). The foldable IOL acts as a barrier to nuclear pieces dropping into the vitreous and works like an artificial posterior capsule. When one haptic is kept out of the incision site, the IOL position can be readily adjusted if the nucleus rotates in the anterior chamber. The chances of IOL drop are also decreased, as the haptic is controlled from the incision (see

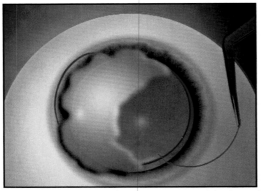

Figure 8-11. Haptic outside the incision can be adjusted so that the optic occludes the pupil.

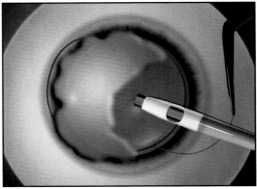

Figure 8-12. Phacoemulsification of the nuclear pieces.

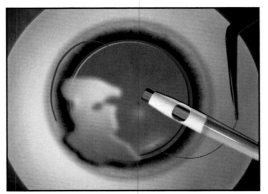

Figure 8-13. IOL acts as a scaffold and prevents the nuclear pieces from falling down.

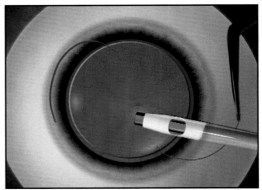

Figure 8-14. Nuclear emulsification complete.

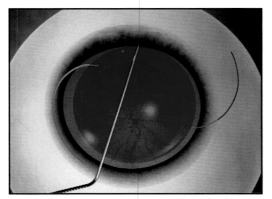

Figure 8-15. IOL repositioning done by shifting the IOL into the sulcus.

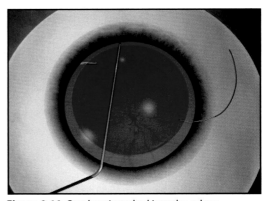

Figure 8-16. One haptic tucked into the sulcus.

Figure 8-12). The presence of the IOL also serves to compartmentalize the eye, which, in turn, decreases hydration of the vitreous from the anterior chamber maintainer and prevents vitreous prolapse into the anterior chamber. Once the nucleus is removed, the same posterior chamber IOL is repositioned into the sulcus (Figure 8-15 to 8-19). As compared to an open wound (after extension), posterior capsular rupture with nonextended phaco incisions are associated with a relatively lower incidence of vitreous loss because the self-sealing, small clear corneal wound provides

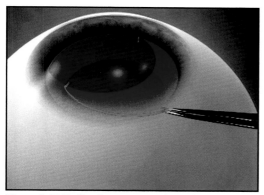

Figure 8-17. Trailing haptic grasped with forceps.

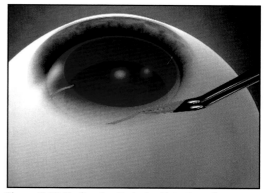

Figure 8-18. Trailing haptic tucked into the sulcus.

Figure 8-19. IOL in the sulcus.

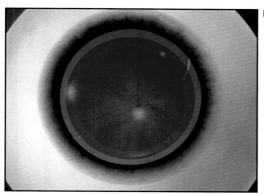

control of ocular integrity. This maintains the anterior chamber and intraocular pressure (IOP) and discourages forward movement of the vitreous, which would occur in the presence of an "open globe" as in ECCE.

GLUED INTRAOCULAR LENS SCAFFOLDING

In certain cases with insufficient iris and anterior capsular support for IOL scaffolding, it may not be prudent to implant the IOL and use it as a scaffold because of the risk of the IOL dropping into the vitreous cavity secondary to lack of support. The authors have been using a technique which they call *glued IOL scaffolding* to provide support during nuclear fragment removal in eyes with insufficient iris support and absent or insufficient capsular support for sulcus placement of the IOL. The authors combine the glued IOL technique and the IOL scaffold technique for glued IOL scaffolding. This situation may be seen in eyes with iris coloboma (Figure 8-20), in which a posterior capsular rupture has occurred and there is no capsular support. It may also be seen in floppy iris syndrome, where the iris is not taut enough to support the IOL, or in cases with non-constricting dilated pupils due to mechanical or surgical trauma, combined with lack of capsular support.

In the event of posterior capsular rupture in these cases, the remaining nuclear pieces are brought to the anterior chamber (Figure 8-21A). An infusion cannula is fixed and scleral flaps are created 180 degrees apart in preparation for glued IOL surgery. A 20-gauge needle then creates a sclerotomy 1 mm behind the limbus under the sclera flaps. A 23-gauge vitrector may be passed through the sclerotomy to perform an anterior vitrectomy (Figure 8-21B). A 3-piece, foldable IOL

Figure 8-20. Iris coloboma with a mature cataract.

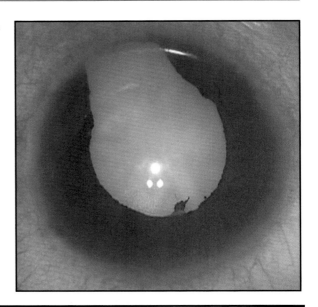

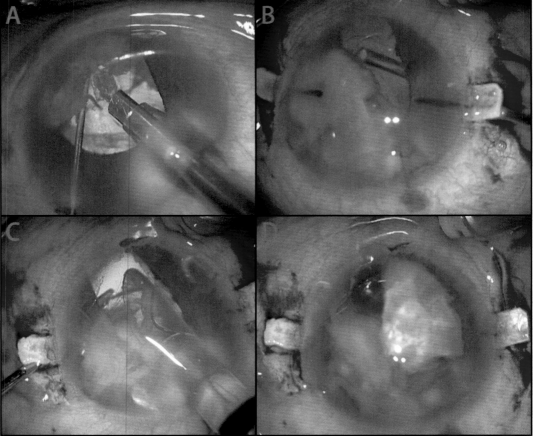

Figure 8-21. Glued IOL scaffold. (A) Phacoemulsification in a mature cataract with iris coloboma. Note the posterior capsular rupture. (B) Preparation for glued IOL surgery. Scleral flaps created. Infusion cannula is fixed. A 23-gauge vitrector may be passed through the sclerotomy to perform an anterior vitrectomy. (C) Three-piece, foldable IOL implantation. Note the cartridge in the anterior chamber. Also note the haptic is slightly out of the cartridge so that it is easy for the glued IOL forceps to grasp the tip of the haptic. Haptic tip grasped with the glued IOL forceps. (D) Both haptics are externalized.

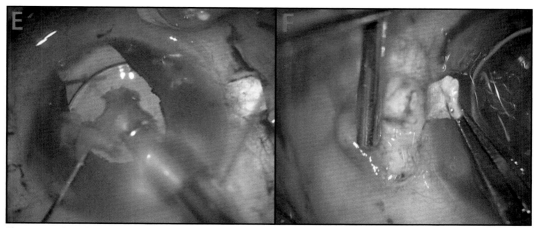

Figure 8-21 (continued). Glued IOL scaffold. (E) Phacoemulsification of the nuclear pieces. Artificial posterior capsule created by the IOL. (F) Fibrin glue application to seal the haptics to the scleral flap.

is loaded into the injector and the cartridge is passed into the anterior chamber (Figure 8-21C). The haptic tip should be left protruding slightly out of the cartridge to allow for easy grasping of the haptic with glued IOL forceps. With the tip of the haptic thus grasped, the IOL is gently injected, while at the same time bringing the cartridge tip out of the main port so that the second haptic trails out of the incision. The risk of the IOL falling down is very low, as the first haptic is caught with the forceps and the second haptic is still trailing outside the clear corneal incision. The second haptic is also subsequently externalized (see Figure 8-9) using the handshake technique (Figure 8-21D). If the nuclear pieces are occupying a significant amount of space in the anterior chamber, implanting the glued IOL in this manner may be difficult. A viscoelastic can be used to dislodge the pieces to the side and gain visualization.

A 26-gauge needle is used to create the intrascleral Scharioth pockets, and the haptics are tucked into the intrascleral pocket. Phacoemulsification of the nuclear pieces is then performed with less risk of fragment drop (Figure 8-21E). Finally, air is injected into the anterior chamber and fibrin glue is used to seal the flaps (Figure 8-21F). An artificial posterior capsule is thus created using the combination of the glued IOL and the IOL scaffold techniques (Figure 8-22).

CONCLUSION

With this IOL scaffolding technique, the IOL acts as a physical barrier to prevent forward movement of the vitreous as well as prevent nuclear fragment drop. Thus, the authors favor this new IOL scaffolding technique in posterior capsular rupture with retained moderate to soft nuclear fragments. However, in cases of hard cataract, conversion to ECCE is ideal. Combining the glued IOL and the IOL scaffold techniques can create an artificial posterior capsule in certain cases of capsular deficiency where the iris is deficient or the pupil is too large to support an IOL for performing an IOL scaffold technique alone.

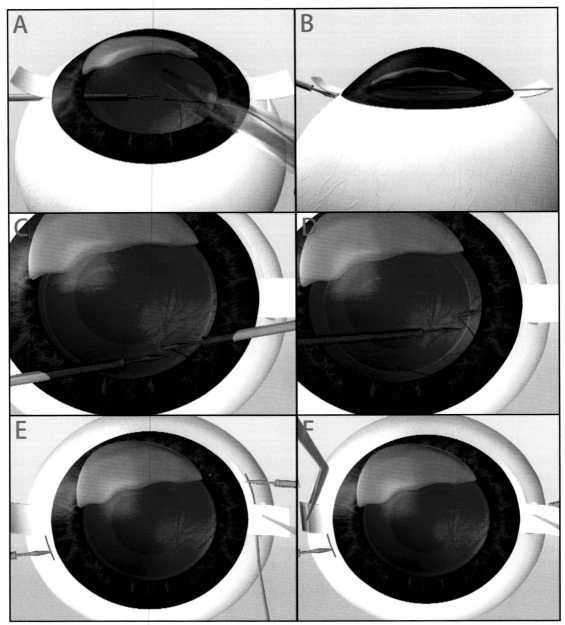

Figure 8-22. Glued IOL scaffold illustrations. (A) Dilated pupil. Nucleus lying in the anterior chamber. Three-piece, foldable IOL injected. Note the sclera flaps are 180 degrees apart and the glued IOL forceps on the left side are ready to grab the haptic of the IOL. (B) Leading haptic externalized. (C) Handshake technique for trailing haptic. (D) Glued IOL forceps catch the trailing haptic tip to externalize. (E) Both haptics externalized. Twenty-six-gauge needle making the Scharioth pocket. (F) Haptic tucked in to the intrascleral pocket on the right. Left side haptic is ready to be tucked.

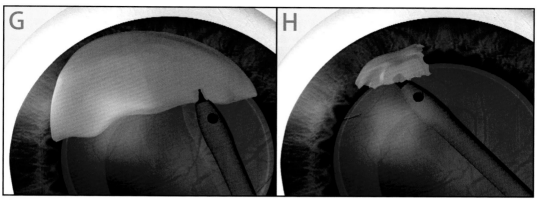

Figure 8-22 (continued). Glued IOL scaffold illustrations. (G) Phacoemulsification of the nuclear piece. The glued IOL now acts as a scaffold. (H) Glued IOL scaffold. Final nuclear piece emulsified. Fibrin glue will then be applied to the scleral flaps.

REFERENCES

1. Vejarano LF, Tello A. Posterior capsular rupture. In: Agarwal A, ed. *Phaco Nightmares; Conquering Cataract Catastrophes.* Thorofare, NJ: SLACK Incorporated; 2006:253-264.
2. Vajpayee RB, Sharma N, Dada T, Gupta V, Kumar A, Dada VK. Management of posterior capsule tears. *Surv Ophthalmol.* 2001;45(6):473-488.
3. Gimbel HV, Sun R, Ferensowicz M, Anderson Penno E, Kamal A. Intraoperative management of posterior capsule tears in phacoemulsification and intraocular lens implantation. *Ophthalmology.* 2001;108(12):2186-2189; discussion 2190-2192.
4. Dada T, Sharma N, Vajpayee RB, Dada VK. Conversion from phacoemulsification to extracapsular cataract extraction: incidence, risk factors, and visual outcome. *J Cataract Refract Surg.* 1998;24(11):1521-1524.
5. Prasad S, Kamath GG. Converting from phacoemulsification to ECCE. *J Cataract Refract Surg.* 1999;25(4):462-463.
6. Thatte S, Raju VK. Phacosandwich technique. *J Cataract Refract Surg.* 1999;25(8):1039-1040.
7. Chang DF, Packard RB. Posterior-assisted levitation for nucleus retrieval using Viscoat after posterior capsule rupture. *J Cataract Refract Surg.* 2003;29(10):1860-1865.
8. Michelson MA. Use of a Sheets' glide as a pseudo-posterior capsule in phacoemulsification complicated by posterior capsule rupture. *Eur J Implant Refract Surg.* 1993;5:70-72.
9. Hansson LJ, Larsson J. Vitrectomy for retained lens fragments in the vitreous after phacoemulsification. *J Cataract Refract Surg.* 2002;28(6):1007-1011.
10. Monshizadeh R, Samiy N, Haimovici R. Management of retained intravitreal lens fragments after cataract surgery. *Surv Ophthalmol.* 1999;43(5):397-404.
11. Kumar DA, Agarwal A, Prakash G, Jacob S, Agarwal A, Sivagnanam S. IOL scaffold technique for posterior capsule rupture. J Refract Surg. 2012;28(5):314-315. doi: 10.3928/1081597X-20120413-01.
12. Agarwal A, Jacob S, Agarwal A, Narasimhan S, Kumar DA, Agarwal A. Glued intraocular lens scaffolding to create an artificial posterior capsule for nucleus removal in eyes with posterior capsule tear and insufficient iris and sulcus support. *J Cataract Refract Surg.* 2013;39(3):326-333. doi: 10.1016/j.jcrs.2013.01.018.
13. Mehta K, Mehta C. Saving the Day: Hema Lifeboat. Eyetube. 2010. Updated May 21, 2010.

III

Intraocular Lens Implantation Strategies in Posterior Capsular Rupture

Iris Claw Intraocular Lens

Marko Ostovic, MD and Thomas Kohnen, MD, PhD, FEBO

Situations such as aphakia, defective posterior capsule,[1-5] or tissue weakness can be challenging for the implantation of an intraocular lens (IOL). A possible procedure for the management of such conditions is the implantation of an iris claw lens. This lens does not need capsular structures for fixation, as the claws of the IOL are fixated onto the iris. The IOL can be implanted retropupillarily or in the anterior chamber. This was first designed by Jan G.F. Worst, MD and popularized by Dr. Daljit Singh.[6]

PREOPERATIVE EXAMINATION

Preoperative examination of the eye is necessary for good postoperative results. Examination parameters should include a complete eye examination, measurement of the intraocular pressure (IOP), endothelial cell count of the cornea, and biometry of the eye including axial length, anterior chamber depth, and keratometry.

SURGICAL TECHNIQUE FOR THE ANTERIOR CHAMBER APPROACH

The following outlines the surgical technique when using the anterior chamber approach:
- Before starting surgery, the pupil should be miotic. This is achieved by applying pilocarpine eye drops just before the actual operation.

Agarwal A.
Posterior Capsular Rupture: A Practical Guide to Prevention and Management (pp 101-104).
© 2014 Taylor & Francis Group.

Figure 9-1. Insertion of the iris claw IOL through a scleral tunnel.

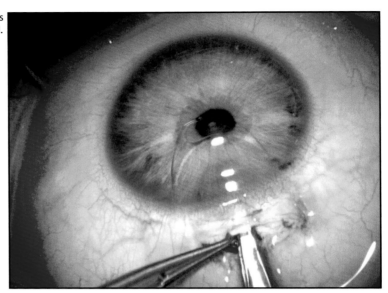

Figure 9-2. Iris claw IOL during surgery. As the surgeon keeps the IOL steady with the right hand instrument, he or she enclavates the second claw into the iris.

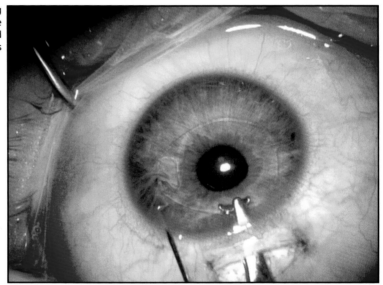

- Preoperative preparation should also include a peripheral iridectomy with the neodymium-doped yttrium aluminum garnet (Nd:YAG) laser or an intraoperative iridectomy with vitrector to avoid high IOP postoperatively.

- A corneal scleral incision or scleral tunnel incision is then created.

- Intraocular pilocarpine is injected to make the pupil miotic, and a vitrector is used to create an iridectomy. A vitrectomy is also performed to clear the vitreous in the anterior chamber. Then, viscoelastics are injected into the anterior chamber.

- The IOL is inserted into the anterior chamber. One may use a spreader device to make the claws spread and capture a particular area of the iris. A needle can also be used for this maneuver. Best overall positions for the claw enclavation are at 3 and 9 o'clock (Figures 9-1 to 9-3).

- Finally, the viscoelastic is removed and, if necessary, sutures are added on the scleral tunnel (Figure 9-4).

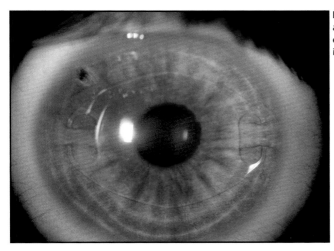

Figure 9-3. Anterior iris claw IOL 1 month after surgery. The lens is centered and the enclavations are both sufficient. Notice the iridectomy at 10 o'clock.

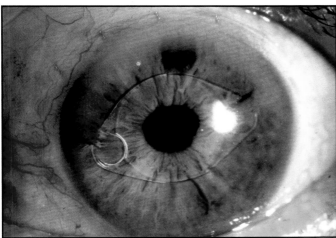

Figure 9-4. Secondary iris claw lens in an intracapsular aphakic patient 15 years postoperatively. (Reprinted with permission from Dr. Ravijit Singh.)

RETROPUPILLARY IMPLANTATION

The following steps should be followed for retropupillary implantation of the iris claw IOL:

- The Artisan lens (Ophtec, Boca Raton, FL) is implanted upside down into the anterior chamber and rotated into a position where the claws can be enclavated into the iris (at 3 and 9 o'clock).
- The lens is then pushed behind the iris.
- A bimanual procedure is performed. With one instrument, the Artisan lens is held in position and, with the spatula, the claws are enclavated into the iris (Figure 9-5).

COMPLICATIONS

This technique is not without complications. When implanting retropupillarily, there always exists the danger of subluxation of the lens in the vitreous body with a resulting expansion of the operation to a vitrectomy. If the implantation is performed in the anterior chamber, the IOL could possibly have contact with the cornea, resulting in endothelial cell loss.[5] Complications, such as uveitis, iris damage, decentration, or loss of enclavation can also occur.

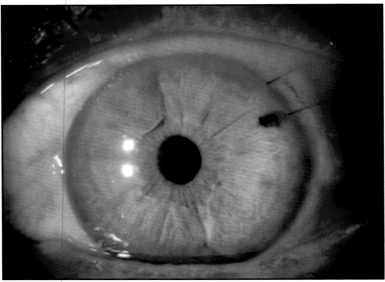

Figure 9-5. Retropupillary iris claw lens implanted. (Reprinted with permission from Dr. Ravijit Singh.)

REFERENCES

1. Agarwal A, Kumar DA, Jacob S, et al. Fibrin glue–assisted sutureless posterior chamber intraocular lens implantation in eyes with deficient posterior capsules. *J Cataract Refract Surg.* 2008;34:1433-1438.
2. Prakash G, Kumar DA, Jacob S, et al. Anterior segment optical coherence tomography–aided diagnosis and primary posterior chamber intraocular lens implantation with fibrin glue in traumatic phacocele with scleral perforation. *J Cataract Refract Surg.* 2009;35:782-784.
3. Prakash G, Jacob S, Kumar DA, et al. Femtosecond-assisted keratoplasty with fibrin glue–assisted sutureless posterior chamber lens implantation: new triple procedure. *J Cataract Refract Surg.* 2009;35:973-979.
4. Agarwal A, Kumar DA, Prakash G, et al. Fibrin glue–assisted sutureless posterior chamber intraocular lens implantation in eyes with deficient posterior capsules [Reply to letter]. *J Cataract Refract Surg.* 2009;35:795-796.
5. Koss MJ, Kohnen T. Intraocular architecture of secondary implanted anterior chamber iris-claw lenses in aphakic eyes evaluated with anterior segment optical coherence tomography. *Br J Ophthalmol.* 2009;93:1301-1306.
6. Fechner PU, Singh D, Wulff K. Iris-claw lens in phasic eyes to correct hyperopia: preliminary study. *J Cataract Refract Surg.* 1998;24:48-56.

Sliding Internal Knot Technique for Late in-the-Bag Intraocular Lens Decentration

Thomas A. Oetting, MS, MD

INTRAOCULAR LENS DISLOCATION

Late dislocation of the intraocular lens (IOL) is an increasingly common problem, especially in patients with pseudoexfoliation.[1,2] Drs. Janet Tsui, Alton Szeto, and this author recently described a technique using a sliding knot for late dislocation, which has been found to be useful for most types of IOLs.[3] This technique is adapted from previously published techniques.[4-10] The sliding internal knot (SLIK) technique has the advantage of an external approach of the needle, with an internal sliding knot that does not require coverage or rotation.

TECHNIQUE

The SLIK technique starts with conjunctiva dissections 180 degrees apart to allow exposure of the sclera in the area of the sulcus close to the location of the IOL haptics. Retracting the iris with a hook may increase exposure of the haptics to ease suturing. A 9-0, double-armed Prolene suture on a long, curved needle (CTC-6L; Ethicon, Cornelia, GA) is passed from the outside through the sclera approximately 1.5 mm posterior to the limbus, passing under the haptic, through the capsular bag and out, avoiding the iris (Figure 10-1). The other needle arm passes just over the haptic, under the iris, and then out through the cornea (Figure 10-2). One side of the suture is pulled with a hook through a paracentesis placed in a location convenient to the surgeon's dominant hand (Figure 10-3). A loop of suture from the other pass of the suture is pulled out through the same paracentesis (Figure 10-4). This leaves a loop and a free end through the same paracentesis, which is similar to the technique described by Siepser[9] for iris repair and Chang[10] for haptic fixation to the iris. The suture loop is wrapped around tying forceps, which in turn grabs the free end of the suture (Figure 10-5). The free end is pulled through the wrapped suture, and then forceps

Agarwal A.
Posterior Capsular Rupture: A Practical Guide to Prevention and Management (pp 105-108).
© 2014 Taylor & Francis Group.

Figure 10-1. Initial pass of the double-armed, 9-0 Prolene suture placed under the haptic and through the capsule.

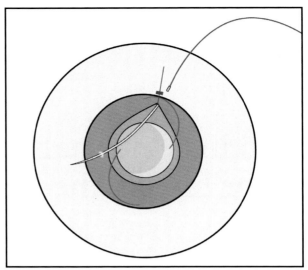

Figure 10-2. Other arm of the 9-0 Prolene suture is passed over the haptic, avoiding the capsule.

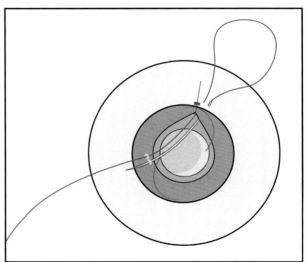

Figure 10-3. One end is pulled completely through the paracentesis.

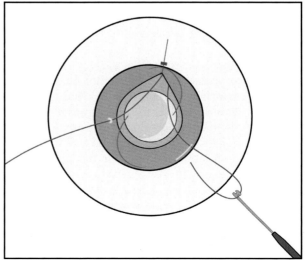

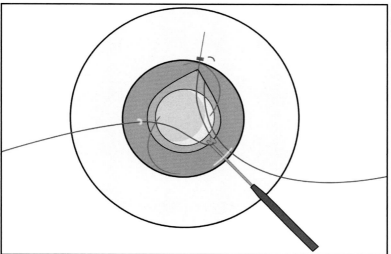

Figure 10-4. The loop from the other end is pulled through the same paracentesis.

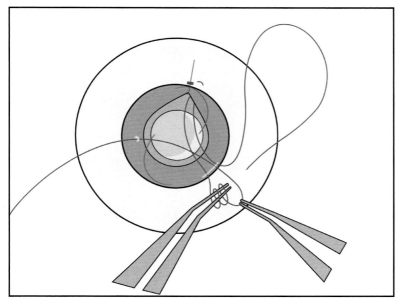

Figure 10-5. Suture from the loop is wrapped around the forceps, and the free end is pulled through and tied using a Siepser sliding knot.

pull the other free end to slip the knot into the anterior chamber (Figure 10-6). Microforceps (Duet; MicroSurgical Technology, Redmond, WA) are used to cinch the knot down snugly to the sclera. Usually, both haptics are tied down to fully secure the IOL. It is very important to cut the suture close to the knot so that the free ends do not irritate the iris.

COMPLICATIONS

The authors described a few complications with the SLIK procedure in a recent review.[3] In 2 patients, vitreous hemorrhage from the scleral passes led to a temporary decline in vision following the procedure, which resolved without intervention.[3] The authors also reported some temporary inflammation from irritation from suture ends that were not cut short enough, and this also resolved with limited intervention.[3] The authors have used this technique on both 3-piece and single-piece acrylic IOLs.

Figure 10-6. Intraocular forceps are used to cinch the knot down to the sclera.

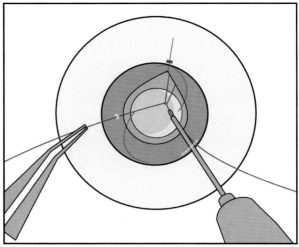

Conclusion

The external approach of the needle passes are easier using SLIK when the IOL is unstable compared with other techniques the authors have tried. In addition, the internal knot eliminates the need for a scleral flap to cover an external knot.

Acknowledgments

The figures have been drawn by the very talented Alton Szeto (www.altonszeto.com).

References

1. Davis D, Brubaker J, Espandar L, et al. Late in-the-bag spontaneous intraocular lens dislocation: evaluation of 86 consecutive cases. *Ophthalmology.* 2009;116(4):664-670.
2. Jakobsson G, Zetterberg M, Lundstrom M, et al. Late dislocation of in-the-bag and out-of-the bag intraocular lenses: ocular and surgical characteristics and time to lens positioning. *J Cataract Refract Surg.* 2010;36:1637-1644.
3. Oetting TA, Tsui JY, Szeto AT. Sliding internal knot technique for late in-the-bag intraocular lens decentration. *J Cataract Refract Surg.* 2011;37(5):810-813.
4. Ahmed II, Chen SH, Kranemann C, Wong DT. Surgical repositioning of dislocated capsular tension rings. *Ophthalmology.* 2005;112:1725-1733.
5. Oshika T. Transscleral suture fixation of a subluxated posterior chamber lens within the capsular bag. *J Cataract Refract Surg.* 1997;23:1421-1424.
6. Hindman HB, Casparis H, Haller JA, Stark WJ. Sutured sulcus fixation of an anteriorly dislocated endocapsular intraocular lens. *Arch Ophthalmol.* 2008;126(11):1567-1570.
7. Hoffman RS, Fine IH, Packer M. Scleral fixation without conjunctival dissection. *J Cataract Refract Surg.* 2006;32:1907-1912.
8. McCannel MA. A retrievable suture idea for anterior uveal problems. *Ophthalmic Surg Lasers.* 1976;7(2):98-103.
9. Siepser SB. The closed chamber slipping suture for iris repair. *Ann Ophthalmol.* 1994;26(3):71-72.
10. Chang DF. Siepser slipknot for McCannel iris-suture fixation of subluxated intraocular lenses. *J Cataract Refract Surg.* 2004;30(6):1170-1176.

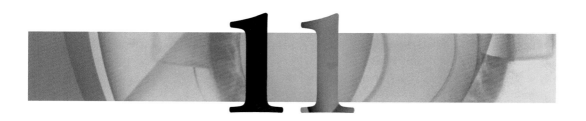

Iris-Fixated Surgical Technique of an Acrylic Intraocular Lens in the Absence of Capsular Support

Yassine Daoud, MD and Walter J. Stark, MD

Inadequate capsular support can be caused by many things. The 3 main reasons for inadequate capsular support are (1) complicated cataract surgery with posterior capsular break or significant zonular loss, (2) result of trauma or secondary to congenital problems (eg, Marfan syndrome, Weill-Marchesani syndrome, homocystinuria, Ehlers-Danlos syndrome, or spherophakia), and (3) secondary to concurrent ocular conditions (eg, pseudoexfoliation).

TREATMENT OPTIONS

Inadequate capsular and zonular support precludes placing an intraocular lens (IOL) into the capsular bag, as it may lead to malpositioning, subluxation, or dislocation of the IOL.

Treatment options include leaving the patient aphakic, placing an open-loop anterior chamber IOL; suture-fixating a 3-piece, foldable acrylic IOL in the ciliary sulcus or the peripheral iris; and sclera fixation in the ciliary sulcus using 10-0 Prolene sutures or glued intrascleral haptic-fixated IOL.

Aphakia may increase the risk of glaucoma and aphakic bullous keratopathy. Beside being cosmetically unacceptable, aphakic spectacles cause significant optical aberrations, limited field of vision, image magnification, and, in cases of unilateral aphakia, anisometropia. Thus, many patients may prefer to wear contact lenses for good visual acuity. However, contact lenses can cause irritation of the cornea, dry eye, and increase the risk of infections and corneal ulcers. In addition, some patients may develop intolerance to the contact lenses. Anterior chamber IOLs may lead to endothelial cell loss, uveitis-glaucoma-hyphema (UGH), pupil distortion, and pseudophakic bullous keratopathy.[1] Anterior chamber IOLs cannot be implanted if there are significant angle abnormalities such as peripheral synechiae. Posteriorly placed IOLs with suturing to the ciliary sulcus can be skill- and time-demanding. Scleral-fixated IOLs may be prone to tilting with subsequent rubbing against the iris, persistent inflammation, segmental angle closure, and possibly

Agarwal A.
Posterior Capsular Rupture: A Practical Guide to Prevention and Management (pp 109-116).
© 2014 Taylor & Francis Group.

UGH.[2,3] In addition, there have been reports of spontaneous subluxation of scleral-fixated IOLs.[4,5] Finally, the transscleral sutures may externalize or erode, potentially causing endophthalmitis.[6]

Suturing the IOL to the peripheral iris using a modified McCannel technique has been shown to be safe, effective, and efficient.[7-10]

PREOPERATIVE EVALUATION

Thorough examination of the anterior chamber is warranted. Special attention should be given to the health of the cornea including any corneal edema, guttae, and, if indicated, endothelial cell count by specular microscopy for proper counseling of the patient. The health of the iris is accessed through direct beam microscopy and retroillumination in an effort to identify any transillumination defects and areas of iris weakness or instability.

INTRAOCULAR LENS TYPES

Single–piece, foldable lenses should be avoided as haptics in the sulcus can cause UGH syndrome. Single-piece, nonfoldable lenses should also be avoided due to the risk of haptic break during the procedure and the potential to develop UGH. Three-piece, foldable lenses are desired for the iris-fixated IOL procedure. The foldable lens allows the procedure to be performed through a small 3.3- to 3.5-mm clear corneal incision, as the haptics are strong enough to help support the sutured IOL. A large lens diameter is desirable to suture the middle of the haptics to the mid-iris. This will encourage some of the haptic to stay in the sutured complex, preventing IOL dislocation in the event of minor haptic slippage. A 6-mm optic has been successfully attempted, but the authors favor a 6.5-mm optic. The authors use the MA50BM 3-piece, acrylic IOL (Alcon Laboratories, Fort Worth, TX). The 6.5-mm optic IOL provides 18% more optic area compared with the 6-mm optic IOL. This is desirable in the rare incidence of pupil abnormality or slight IOL decentration. The larger optic will still be able to cover the pupillary axis and prevent diplopia. An aspheric IOL is not recommended to minimize the optical aberrations that may occur with IOL decentration. In eyes with no capsular support, the authors prefer inserting the IOL by using folding forceps, rather than using a plunger or twist-injection mechanism. This affords finer control of the IOL and allows for better positioning and "pupillary capture" of the IOL haptics in preparation for the procedure. Prior to the surgery, pharmacological pupillary dilation should be avoided if possible so the pupil can be constricted around the haptic optic junction prior to suture placement. If pupillary dilatation is necessary, it can be achieved with a retrobulbar anesthesia injection.

INTRAOPERATIVE PREPARATION PRIOR TO IRIS FIXATION OF THE INTRAOCULAR LENS

Complicated Cataract Surgery

In the case of complicated cataract surgery, it is important to ensure that as much of the lens material is removed as possible. A thorough and adequate anterior or pars plana vitrectomy should ensue.

Secondary Intraocular Lens

Thorough inspection of the anterior chamber should be carried out to check for any vitreous in the anterior chamber. This can be achieved by using intravitreal triamcinolone acetonide (Kenalog) in the anterior chamber and then washing it out. Kenalog stains and aids in visualizing vitreous strands that otherwise may not be seen. Alternatively, placing air in the anterior chamber will help identify vitreous strands that may be missed.

Subluxed Intraocular Lens

Initially, if the subluxed IOL is a single-piece acrylic lens, it will have to be removed. A 3.5-mm clear corneal incision is created. Viscoelastic material is injected into the anterior chamber to help protect the corneal endothelial cells. The subluxed IOL is brought to the anterior chamber. With a Barraquer sweep and IOL inserter, the IOL is folded and removed from the eye. Alternative methods may include cutting the IOL and removing the pieces individually. If there is vitreous prolapse, a core anterior or pars plana vitrectomy may be performed.

If the subluxed lens is a 3-piece IOL, it can be brought to the anterior chamber using the method described in the following section.

Dislocated Intraocular Lens Into the Vitreous Cavity

If the IOL is dislocated into the vitreous cavity, a pars plana vitrectomy (typically done by a vitreoretinal specialist) should be performed, with special attention to hidden breaks or tears in the retina. The IOL optic should be brought to the AC. If the dislocated IOL is a single piece, it will have to be removed. If it is a 3-piece IOL with good nonmalformed haptics, then it may be used for the iris-suturing procedure. The IOL should be brought to the anterior chamber in such a way that the optic is in front of the iris plane and the haptics are behind the iris plane (pupillary capture).

IRIS SUTURING PROCEDURE

The pupil is constricted with acetylcholine to facilitate pupillary capture of the IOL optic. Viscoelastic material is injected to deepen the anterior chamber. The IOL is folded in a "moustache" fold and inserted through the corneal wound (Figure 11-1A). Care must be taken not to bend or break the trailing haptic in this process. To do so, the trailing haptic may need to be individually inserted with the help of insertion forceps (Figure 11-1B). The haptics should be placed within the sulcus and the optic should be above the plane of the iris (Figure 11-1C). A Barraquer sweep is passed through the paracentesis and placed beneath the optic as the lens is unfolded to ensure pupillary capture (Figures 11-1D to 11-1F). Additional viscoelastic material is injected into the anterior chamber. The optic is then elevated with the Barraquer sweep so that the haptics contour is visualized through the iris, simplifying passage of the sutures. Using a modified McCannel-type iris-fixation technique, a 10-0 Prolene suture is passed on a needle (CTC-6; Ethicon, Bridgewater, NJ) through clear cornea and the iris, under the peripheral aspect of the first haptic, then out through the iris and clear cornea (Figure 11-2A). It is important to pass the suture through the iris in the periphery where there is a significant area of iris redundancy. As little iris as possible should be involved in the suture. The authors avoid placing the suture close to the pupillary border, which could result in pupil ovalization. A paracentesis is created over the first haptic and the 2 ends of the suture are pulled through this site. Care must be taken to ensure that both ends of the suture exit from the same paracentesis wound without corneal tissue incarceration by the sutures (Figure 11-2B). The second haptic is secured in a similar manner, making sure the sutures are 180 degrees apart (Figure 11-2C). The sutures are tied with a locking 3-1-1 throw.

Figure 11-1. (A) The IOL is bent into a "moustache" fold. (B) The trailing haptic may need to be individually inserted with the help of insertion forceps to avoid haptic breakage. (C) The haptics should be placed within the sulcus and the optic should be above the plane of the iris. (Reprinted with permission from Stutzman RD, Stark WJ. Surgical technique for suture fixation of an acrylic intraocular lens in the absence of capsular support. *J Cataract Refract Surg.* 2003;29(9):1658-1662.)

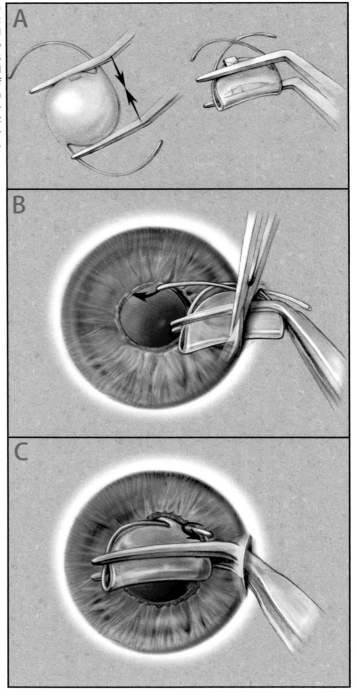

The optic is placed posterior to the iris (Figure 11-2D). If there is no remaining capsular support, the sutures are tied tightly before the IOL optic is placed into the posterior chamber. If there is no prior vitrectomy, the remaining capsule and the vitreous base can be used to help support the lens. In this case, after externalizing the suture ends, a 3-knot is created to secure a haptic to the iris. This is repeated for the second haptic. Then, the optic is placed posterior to the iris using a

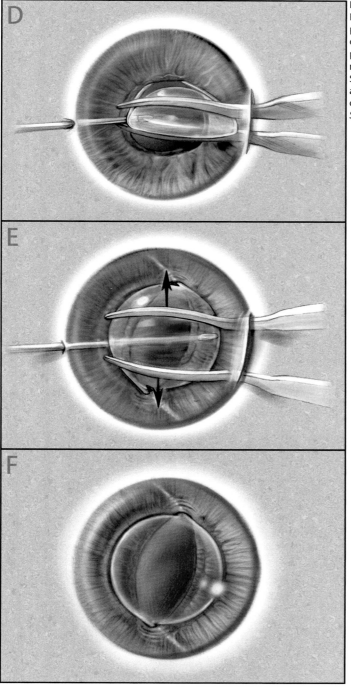

Figure 11-1 (continued). (D-F) A Barraquer sweep is passed through the paracentesis and placed beneath the optic as the lens is unfolded to ensure pupillary capture. (Reprinted with permission from Stutzman RD, Stark WJ. Surgical technique for suture fixation of an acrylic intraocular lens in the absence of capsular support. *J Cataract Refract Surg.* 2003;29(9):1658-1662.)

Sinskey hook (see Figure 11-2D). After the IOL is adequately centered, each knot can be finished and secured with an additional 1-1 throw.

Using a Sinskey hook, the iris is manipulated to produce a round pupil (see Figure 11-2D). Acetylcholine chloride is injected again to ensure a round miotic pupil (Figure 11-3). The retained viscoelastic material is removed from the anterior chamber.

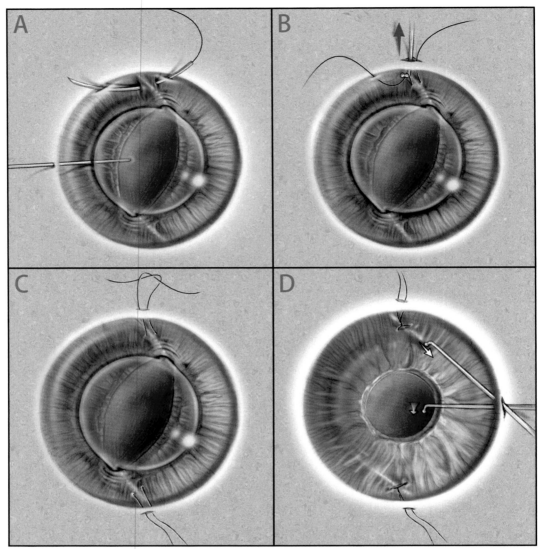

Figure 11-2. (A) A 10-0 polypropylene suture is passed on a needle through clear cornea and the iris and is placed under the peripheral aspect of the first haptic, then out through the iris and clear cornea. (B) Care must be taken to ensure that both ends of the suture exit from the same paracentesis wound without corneal tissue incarceration by the sutures. (C) The second haptic is secured in a similar manner as shown in Figure 11-3, making sure the sutures are 180 degrees apart. The sutures are tied with a locking 3-1-1 throw. (D) The optic is placed posterior to the iris using a Sinskey hook. The iris is manipulated to produce a round pupil. (Reprinted with permission from Stutzman RD, Stark WJ. Surgical technique for suture fixation of an acrylic intraocular lens in the absence of capsular support. *J Cataract Refract Surg.* 2003;29(9):1658-1662.)

Air is injected into the anterior chamber and checked for unidentified strands of vitreous. If vitreous is present, a Barraquer sweep is used to break the strands, or a more extensive vitrectomy is performed. Then, a repeat injection of air is made into the anterior chamber, again inspecting for vitreous. All viscoelastic should be removed from the anterior chamber. A balanced salt solution is injected into the anterior chamber, bringing the eye to physiologic pressure. A 10-0 nylon suture is used to close the main corneal wound. The sideports, as well as the main incision, are hydrated and tested for leaks. Pars plana vitrectomy is often performed with infusion in the anterior chamber and the vitrectomy cutter in the vitreous cavity. This ensures that all vitreous in the anterior chamber will be pushed into the posterior chamber where it is excised using the vitreous cutter.

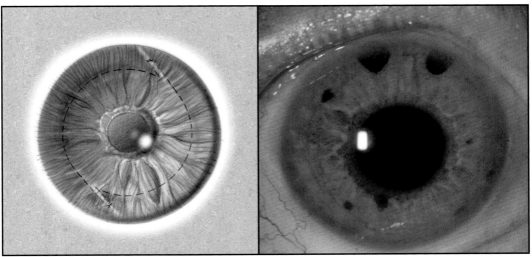

Figure 11-3. Acetylcholine is injected to ensure a round miotic pupil. (Reprinted with permission from Stutzman RD, Stark WJ. Surgical technique for suture fixation of an acrylic intraocular lens in the absence of capsular support. *J Cataract Refract Surg*. 2003;29(9):1658-1662.)

SURGICAL PEARLS FOR IRIS FIXATION OF AN INTRAOCULAR LENS

The following is a list of surgical pearls for iris fixation:

- Pass a Barraquer sweep through the paracentesis and place it beneath the optic as the lens is unfolded to ensure pupillary capture and to prevent IOL dislocation to the vitreous cavity.

- Using a Barraquer sweep, lift the optic to better visualize the contour of the haptics for easy suture passage.

- Use a 10-0 Prolene suture, which does not biodegrade. However, do not place the suture in the haptic eyelet, as sharp edges of the eyelet can mechanically cut the suture over an 8- to 10-year period.

- Pass the suture approximately 1 mm in clear cornea for easy suture visualization and retrieval. Do not pass the suture at the surgical limbus or in the angle.

- Pass the suture in the iris periphery to avoid pupil ovalization.

- Manipulate the iris with a Sinskey hook to produce a round pupil before securing the knots.

Advantages

The following is a list of advantages of iris fixation of an IOL:

- No need for specialized lenses
- Efficient
- Small clear corneal incision (3.3 to 3.5 mm)
- No significant induced astigmatism
- No suture-related problems (eg, erosion, abscess, endophthalmitis)
- No UGH
- Less technically challenging than a scleral-fixated IOL
- Longer longevity than a scleral-fixated IOL

- Conjunctival preservation (in case of possible future surgery)
- Can be performed concurrently with other procedures (Descemet stripping automated endothelial keratoplasty)
- Can be done in the presence of a bleb or glaucoma-drainage device

Disadvantages

The following is a list of disadvantages of performing iris fixation of an IOL:

- Moderate learning curve
- Cannot be used in eyes with significant iris trauma or damage
- May lead to irregular pupil shape if the IOL is sutured near the pupillary margin
- Intraoperatively, the IOL may dislocate posteriorly if proper optic capture is not present

Contraindications

Contraindications of performing iris fixation of an IOL are severe iris atrophy and significant disruption of the anterior segment from trauma or congenital anomalies.

CONCLUSION

In eyes without capsular support, this iris fixation of an IOL technique has been shown to be safe and effective with significant improvement in visual acuity and reduction in refractive error. During a mean follow-up period of 1.5 years, only minimal, transient, and reversible side effects occurred.[11] This technique permits the surgeon to properly treat patients who develop loss of capsule support at the time of cataract surgery and facilitates the management of IOL problems after surgery that require IOL exchange. It also allows secondary IOL insertion in aphakic patients who are contact lens intolerant. The authors prefer this technique in all patients, except for those who have significant loss, instability, or trauma to the iris. In such patients, a scleral-fixated IOL would be the appropriate choice.

REFERENCES

1. Evereklioglu C, Er H, Bekir NA, et al. Comparison of secondary implantation of flexible open-loop anterior chamber and scleral-fixated posterior chamber intraocular lenses. *J Cataract Refract Surg.* 2003;29(2):301-308.
2. Por YM, Lavin MJ. Techniques of intraocular lens suspension in the absence of capsular/zonular support. *Surv Ophthalmol.* 2005;50:429-462.
3. Manabe S-I, Oh H, Amino K, et al. Ultrasound biomicroscopic analysis of posterior chamber intraocular lenses with transscleral sulcus suture. *Ophthalmology.* 2000;107:2172-2178.
4. Assia EI, Nemet A, Sachs D. Bilateral spontaneous subluxation of scleral-fixated intraocular lenses. *J Cataract Refract Surg.* 2002;28(12):2214-2216.
5. Kim J, Kinyoun JL, Saperstein DA, Porter SL. Subluxation of transscleral sutured posterior chamber intraocular lens (TSIOL). *Am J Ophthalmol.* 2003;136(2):382-384.
6. Schechter RJ. Suture-wick endophthalmitis with sutured posterior chamber intraocular lenses. *J Cataract Refract Surg.* 1990;16(6):755-756.
7. McCannel MA. A retrievable suture idea for anterior uveal problems. *Ophthalmic Surg.* 1976;7(2):98-103.
8. Stark WJ, Michels RG, Bruner WE. Management of posteriorly dislocated intraocular lenses. *Ophthalmic Surg.* 1980;11:495-497.
9. Stark WJ, Goodman G, Goodman D, Gottsch J. Posterior chamber intraocular lens implantation in the absence of posterior capsular support. *Ophthalmic Surg.* 1988;19:240-243.
10. Stutzman RD, Stark WJ. Surgical technique for suture fixation of an acrylic intraocular lens in the absence of capsule support. *J Cataract Refract. Surg.* 2003;29:1658-1662.
11. Condon GP, Masket S, Kranemann C, Crandall AS, Ahmed IK. Small-incision iris fixation of foldable intraocular lenses in the absence of capsule support. *Ophthalmology.* 2007;114(7):1311-1318.

Iridal and Scleral-Sutured Intraocular Lenses

Brian C. Stagg, MD; Bryce R. Radmall, MD; and Balamurali Krishna Ambati, MD, PhD

Although innumerable advances, improvements, and discoveries have been made in the discipline of cataract surgery since Dr. Harold Ridley[1,2] implanted the first permanent lens into the human eye 60 years ago, it is still preferable to place the prosthetic lens into the capsular bag, if possible. However, there are many circumstances that prohibit an ophthalmic surgeon's placement of an intraocular lens (IOL) into the capsule. Such circumstances include preexisting conditions resulting in subluxation of the native lens such as Marfan syndrome (Figure 12-1), homocystinuria, surgical complications, and trauma. Severe infections, endophthalmitis, and uveitis can also compromise capsular integrity. These conditions necessitate a novel approach to IOL fixation.

A logical approach to IOL fixation is to attach it in place using sutures. This is commonly performed by suturing the IOL to either the iris or the sclera. A review from the American Academy of Ophthalmology (AAO) demonstrated that both iris-sutured posterior chamber IOLs and scleral-sutured posterior chamber IOLs are safe and effective options for IOL fixation in an eye that lacks capsular support.[3]

IRIS-SUTURED INTRAOCULAR LENS

Although various methods of IOL fixation have proven to be safe and effective, each situation dictates which method is best to use and each differs in technical demand, intraoperative time, structural prerequisite, and associated surgical complications. Indications, methods, prognosis/outcomes, and complications pertaining to iris-sutured IOLs will be discussed.

Agarwal A.
Posterior Capsular Rupture: A Practical Guide to Prevention and Management (pp 117-126).
© 2014 Taylor & Francis Group.

Figure 12-1. Subluxated crystalline lens due to Marfan syndrome. (Reprinted with permission from Dr. Agarwal's Eye Hospital, Chennai, India.)

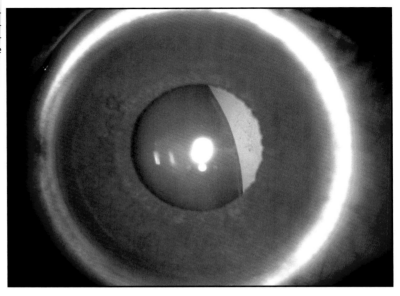

Indications

Iris-sutured IOLs are located away from the trabecular meshwork, which helps to avoid injury to the angle structures, decreases associated inflammation, and reduces suture exposure risk.[4] In addition, the advent of foldable IOLs, smaller incisions, and a new iris-suturing technique has resulted in increased enthusiasm and popularity for utilization of the iris-sutured posterior chamber IOL.[4-9] Furthermore, a posterior chamber IOL theoretically causes less irritation to the cornea, iris, and angle structures, thereby reducing the chances of corneal decompensation or glaucoma when compared to an anterior chamber IOL.[10,11] Thus, a younger patient with healthy iris tissue may better tolerate an iris-sutured IOL long-term.[12]

Sufficient iris tissue to support the lens is requisite when fixating a posterior chamber IOL to the iris; consequently, similar to anterior chamber IOLs, iris-sutured posterior chamber IOLs cannot be used in the setting of marked iris tissue loss, atrophy, or instability.[12] An iris-sutured posterior chamber IOLs would be a poor choice in the setting of trauma to the iris (Figure 12-2). When indicated, iris fixation of a posterior chamber IOL can be an excellent choice, as it offers the benefits of posterior chamber positioning and it is generally thought to be less technically demanding when compared with scleral fixation.

Methods

This section will provide a brief review of the methods and techniques for proper placement of an iris-sutured posterior chamber IOL. A detailed, step-by-step description is available in the literature.[3] Placement of an iris-sutured posterior chamber IOL was first described by McCannel[13] in 1976 by using a limbal incision and stabilizing the posterior chamber IOL by suturing the iris to the haptics. This is performed by first making paracenteses at the 3- and 9-o'clock positions, followed by removal of any vitreous that may be present in the anterior chamber. The posterior chamber IOL is then inserted through a main incision at 12 o'clock. Each haptic is secured by passing a 10-0 polypropylene suture through the peripheral cornea, iris, around the haptic, and back through the iris and cornea. After securing each haptic, the optic is readjusted to assure its proper positioning posterior to the iris. Alternatively, a posterior chamber IOL may be fixated to the iris by suturing the optic itself to the iris rather than tethering it to the haptic.[14]

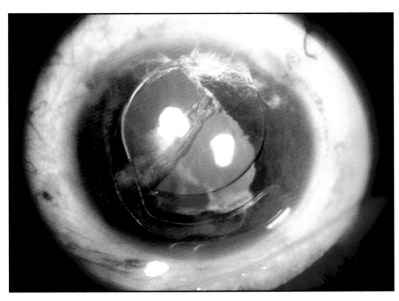

Figure 12-2. Anterior chamber IOL. (Reprinted with permission from Dr. Agarwal's Eye Hospital, Chennai, India.)

In special cases where concomitant penetrating keratoplasty is to be performed, it is possible to perform iris-sutured posterior chamber IOL placement in an open-sky fashion. There are various techniques of iris fixation in an open sky situation, one of which utilizes an optic with 4 holes for the passage of the suture[15] and another that describes a similar approach where the needle is driven directly through the optic itself.[16]

Prognosis/Outcomes

Iris-sutured posterior chamber IOLs have consistently demonstrated safety and efficacy with regard to visual outcome over several series when compared to anterior chamber IOLs and scleral-sutured posterior chamber IOLs.[1,9,16-18] Because the iris-sutured technique places the IOL in the posterior chamber, iris-sutured posterior chamber IOLs are located both near the nodal point of the eye and the eye's rotational axis.[4] This positioning provides a theoretic advantage when compared with anterior chamber IOLs for achieving the best possible visual outcome, although a prospective study of patients with Marfan syndrome-associated lens subluxation demonstrated no difference in visual outcomes at 1 year when comparing iris-sutured posterior chamber IOLs to iris-claw anterior chamber IOLs.[19]

A possible benefit of iris-sutured posterior chamber IOL—when compared with the scleral-sutured approach—is that peripheral iris support does not require blind transscleral-suture passes nor an externalized suture; however, most of these series utilized an open-sky approach, which is technically less challenging than a limbal approach.[3,9,16,17] The only prospective randomized study comparing anterior chamber IOLs, scleral-attached posterior chamber IOLs, and iris-attached posterior chamber IOLs in the setting of penetrating keratoplasty showed that iris-fixated IOLs demonstrated a statistically significant decrease in the risk of complications (cystoid macular edema [CME]), although no difference in visual acuity across the groups was detected.[1]

Complications

Some of the potential complications associated with sutured iris fixation result from disruption of the iris architecture, which can lead to peripheral anterior synechiae, dyscoria, and limitation in the physiologic function of the iris (inability to appropriately dilate).[4,19] As complete dilation may become problematic, it is not ideal to implant an iris-sutured posterior chamber IOL in a patient with significant retinal comorbidities, such as diabetic retinopathy, that will require serial monitoring with the need for adequate fundus visualization. Iridodialysis has been reported with peripheral placement of sutures.[7] Risk of hemorrhage during needle passage is relatively low when the sutures are correctly positioned in the midperipheral iris. The major arterial circle is positioned away from the site of the suture at the root of the iris, and the suture site contains only small diameter, encapsulated vessels.[19] Erosion of an iris suture into an adjacent vessel has also been reported to result in transient hyphema.[7]

Iris chafe and chronic uveitis are additional complications associated with suture placement within the iris and may lead to chronic inflammation as the iris moves to allow for repetitive pupillary dilation and constriction. Mild to moderate local inflammation has been noted in some iris-sutured posterior chamber IOLs.[20] Location and tightness of the suture have also proven to be paramount. As the central iris is most mobile, a suture that is placed too centrally can result in excessive inflammation.[4] A suture that is too tight or travels too far into the iris tissue causes distortion and peaking of the pupil.

It is also important to remember that an iris-sutured IOL is susceptible to complications common to all types of posterior chamber IOLs including CME (Figure 12-3), endophthalmitis, hyphema, vitreous hemorrhage, suprachoroidal hemorrhage (Figure 12-4), and retinal detachment.[4]

SCLERAL-SUTURED INTRAOCULAR LENSES

Using sutures to fixate implanted IOLs to the sclera is a commonly used method to stabilize the IOL in the situation of poor capsular support. A distinct advantage of this method is that the IOL is in the posterior chamber, in a location close to the natural position of the lens. This allows for an appropriate distance from the corneal endothelium and trabecular meshwork, in addition to providing excellent optical correction.

In 1986, Malbran et al[21] presented an early paper describing the technique of suture-fixated IOL implantation in the setting of poor capsular support. Since that time, many modifications and advances have been made to the original technique. Techniques for scleral-sutured fixation can be divided into 2 basic categories: ab externo and ab interno methods. The fundamental difference is that with ab externo methods, the suture is passed from the exterior of the eye to the inside, whereas with ab interno methods, the suture is passed from the interior to the exterior of the eye.

Indications

The basic indication for scleral-sutured IOL placement is the same as for any other form of IOL fixation—lack of capsular support. This occurs when the capsule is weakened due to either damage or intrinsic weakness resulting from a disease process. Scleral-sutured fixation has been used in many situations including pseudoexfoliation (Figure 12-5), Marfan syndrome, traumatic aphakia, and penetrating ocular trauma.[22-25]

One of the primary reasons to choose scleral-sutured IOL placement rather than anterior chamber placement of the IOL is to avoid damage to the corneal endothelium or trabecular meshwork, particularly in patients that are susceptible to these problems. Examples include patients with shallow anterior depth or previous damage to the corneal endothelium. It has also been suggested that scleral-sutured IOLs may be preferred in patients with Marfan syndrome because of the anatomy of the anterior chamber.[24] The major concerns that cause surgeons to favor the use of an anterior chamber IOL over scleral fixation are longer surgical time and increased technical difficulty.

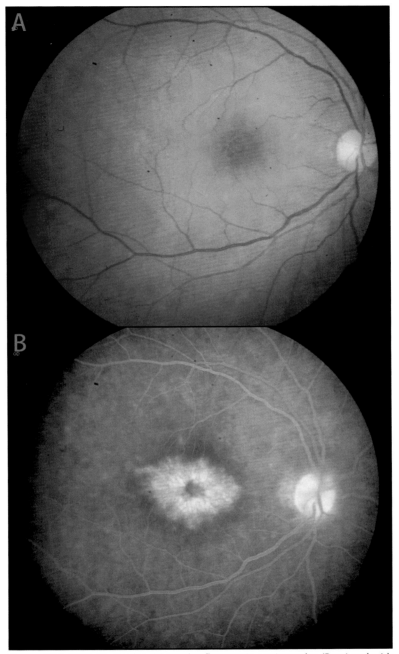

Figure 12-3. CME. (A) Fundus. (B) Fundus fluorescein angiography. (Reprinted with permission from Dr. Agarwal's Eye Hospital, Chennai, India.)

Figure 12-4. Rupture of a ciliary vessel. (A) The normal ciliary vasculature. (B) An aneurysm or swelling of one of the vessels is visible. (C) One of the swollen vessels ruptured, leading to an expulsive hemorrhage. (Reprinted with permission from Dr. Agarwal's Eye Hospital, Chennai, India.)

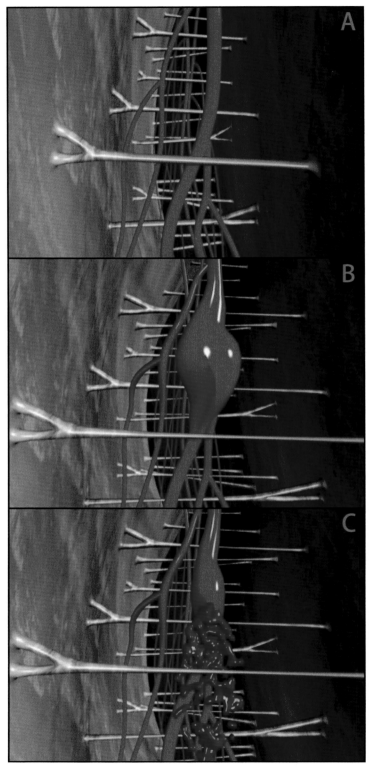

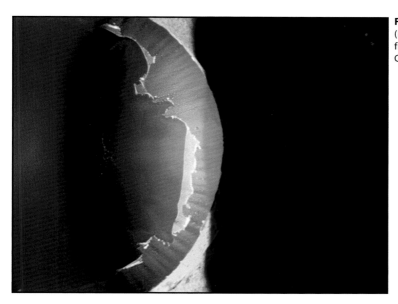

Figure 12-5. Pseudoexfoliation. (Reprinted with permission from Dr. Agarwal's Eye Hospital, Chennai, India.)

Method

Scleral-sutured IOL fixation is often used to anchor newly placed IOLs. Correct placement of the IOL in the posterior chamber with the haptics in the sulcus is of vital importance in the scleral-sutured method. Identification of the ciliary sulcus for lens placement has been performed using various techniques. The most common method uses external landmarks, usually the distance from the limbus. However, intraocular endoscopy, ultrasonography, and transillumination have also been used.[26-28]

Sutured scleral fixation most commonly employs double-armed Prolene polypropylene sutures sized 8–0, 9–0, or 10–0. Polyester (Mersilene), polyethylene (Novafil), or polytetrafluoroethylene (GORE-TEX) are other suture materials that have been used. Techniques using both straight (STC-6) and curved needles (CIF-4 or CTC-6) have been described (Ethicon, Somerville, NJ). Straight needles provide longer range of access, whereas curved needles provide more needle rigidity.

Foldable lens forceps are commonly used for implantation of scleral-sutured IOLs because they allow the haptics of the lens to be dialed during implantation. Recent articles have described using injection systems to place the IOL for scleral-sutured fixation.[29,30] Suggested advantages to using injection systems include smaller incisions, decreased surgical trauma, and maintenance of intraocular pressure (IOP) during the procedure.[29]

To provide access to the ciliary sulcus, conceal the knot, and prevent suture erosion, scleral grooves,[31,32] tunnels,[33,34] or flaps[29,35,36] are created. An important limitation of these techniques is they require extremely accurate suture placement. To combat this difficulty, hollow needles are frequently used as docking guides to ensure exit of the suture needle through the appropriate location.[34,36] Some methods eliminate the need to conceal a fixation knot by utilizing internally tightening sliding knots.[37] Others methods avoid conjunctival dissection.[33]

One-point,[38] 2-point,[21] 3-point, and 4-point[31] scleral-sutured fixation techniques have been described in the literature. Some techniques describe tying knots directly to the haptic,[30,36] although IOLs have been developed with eyelets on the haptics to aid in sutured fixation and prevent slippage of the knots. Some authors suggest temporary haptic externalization for suture placement; suggested advantages of this approach include easy creation of suture loop and stabilization of the IOL.[30]

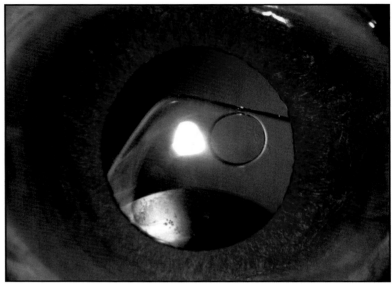

Figure 12-6. Subluxated plate haptic IOL. (Reprinted with permission from Dr. Agarwal's Eye Hospital, Chennai, India.)

Dislocated IOLs (Figure 12-6) that were initially implanted into the capsular bag can be repositioned and fixated using the scleral suture technique without requiring explanation. If the IOL remains within the bag and the IOL-capsular bag complex has dislocated, the entire complex can be fixated using scleral sutures. A sliding Siepser knot is often used in these situations.[36,37]

Prognosis

The prognosis and outcome for patients receiving scleral-sutured IOL fixation is generally very good. A review of recent case series suggests that the majority of patients will experience improved visual acuity. Patients with ocular comorbidities are more likely to experience less desirable outcomes. Zhen et al[24] found similar outcomes between scleral-fixated and iris-fixated IOLs, and both were considered successful.[24] Several important indicators for prognosis after scleral-sutured IOL fixation are minimization of IOL tilt, centration of the IOL, correct location of IOL haptics, and concealment of the knot to avoid erosion.[32-34]

Complications

The introduction of a foreign object to the eye, such as a suture, brings with it certain risks. Two risks that are directly related to the placement of the suture are suture erosion and endophthalmitis. Both can be reduced by burying or concealing the suture.[31] There are also possible complications related to the IOL itself, including IOL tilt, decentration, and dislocation.[26,31,32] As scleral-sutured IOL placement involves full-thickness penetration of the eye, it poses several significant possible complications including ciliary bleeding, vitreous hemorrhage, subconjunctival hemorrhage, and retinal detachment.[31,35,39] Although these complications are relatively rare, they do pose a significant threat. Risk of retinal detachment or intraocular hemorrhage is higher in myopes, hypertensives, or patients taking anticoagulants. A distinct advantage of scleral-sutured IOLs is that they avoid some of the significant risks associated with anterior chamber IOLs including pupillary block, chronic corneal endothelial damage, and damage to the angle.

REFERENCES

1. Por YM, Lavin MJ. Techniques of intraocular lens suspension in the absence of capsular/zonular support. *Surv Ophthalmol.* 2005;50:429-462. doi:10.1016/j.survophthal.2005.06.010
2. Apple DJ, Mamalis N, Loftfield K, et al. Complications of intraocular lenses. A historical and histopathological review. *Surv Ophthalmol.* 1984;29(1):1-54. Review.
3. Wagoner MD, Cox TA, Ariyasu RG, Jacobs DS, Karp CL. Intraocular lens implantation in the absence of capsular support: a report by the American Academy of Ophthalmology. *Ophthalmology.* 2003;110:840-859.
4. Schein OD, Kenyon KR, Steinert RF, et al. A randomized trial of intraocular lens fixation techniques with penetrating keratoplasty. *Ophthalmology.* 1993;100:1437-1443.
5. Mura JJ, Pavlin CJ, Condon GP, et al. Ultrasound biomicroscopic analysis of iris-sutured foldable posterior chamber intraocular lenses. *Am J Ophthalmol.* 2010;149:245-252 e242. doi:10.1016/j.ajo.2009.08.022
6. Condon GP. Simplified small-incision peripheral iris fixation of an AcrySof intraocular lens in the absence of capsule support. *J Cataract Refract Surg.* 2003;29:1663-1667.
7. Michaeli A, Assia EI. Scleral and iris fixation of posterior chamber lenses in the absence of capsular support. *Curr Opin Ophthalmol.* 2005;16:57-60.
8. Stutzman RD, Stark WJ. Surgical technique for suture fixation of an acrylic intraocular lens in the absence of capsule support. *J Cataract Refract Surg* 2003;29:1658-1662.
9. Condon GP, Masket S, Kranemann C, Crandall AS, Ahmed, II. Small-incision iris fixation of foldable intraocular lenses in the absence of capsule support. *Ophthalmology.* 2007;114:1311-1318. doi:10.1016/j.ophtha.2007.04.018
10. Solomon K, Gussler JR, Gussler C, Van Meter WS. Incidence and management of complications of transsclerally sutured posterior chamber lenses. *J Cataract Refract Surg.* 1993;19:488-493.
11. Apple DJ, Price FW, Gwin T, et al. Sutured retropupillary posterior chamber intraocular lenses for exchange or secondary implantation. The 12th annual Binkhorst lecture, 1988. *Ophthalmology.* 1989;96:1241-1247.
12. Boerman H, Chu Y. IOL Implantation without capsular support. *Cataract and Refractive Surgery Today.* 2006(5):23-26.
13. McCannel MA. A retrievable suture idea for anterior uveal problems. *Ophthalmic Surg.* 1976;7:98-103.
14. Navia-Aray EA. Suturing a posterior chamber intraocular lens to the iris through limbal incisions: results in 30 eyes. *J Refract Corneal Surg.* 1994;10:565-570.
15. Soong HK, Musch DC, Kowal V, Sugar A, Meyer RF. Implantation of posterior chamber intraocular lenses in the absence of lens capsule during penetrating keratoplasty. *Arch Ophthalmol.* 1989;107:660-665.
16. Zeh WG, Price FW Jr. Iris fixation of posterior chamber intraocular lenses. *J Cataract Refract Surg.* 2000;26:1028-1034.
17. Akpek EK, Altan-Yaycioglu R, Karadayi K, Christen W, Stark WJ. Long-term outcomes of combined penetrating keratoplasty with iris-sutured intraocular lens implantation. *Ophthalmology.* 2003;110:1017-1022. doi:10.1016/S0161-6420(03)00097-6
18. Farjo AA, Rhee DJ, Soong HK, Meyer RF, Sugar A. Iris-sutured posterior chamber intraocular lens implantation during penetrating keratoplasty. *Cornea.* 2004;23:18-28.
19. Hirashima DE, Soriano ES, Meirelles RL, Alberti GN, Nose W. Outcomes of iris-claw anterior chamber versus iris-fixated foldable intraocular lens in subluxated lens secondary to Marfan syndrome. *Ophthalmology.* 2010;117:1479-1485. doi:10.1016/j.ophtha.2009.12.043
20. Cameron J, Apple D, Sumsion M. Pathology of iris support intraocular lenses. *Implant.* 1987;6:15-24.
21. Malbran ES, Malbran E Jr, Negri I. Lens guide suture for transport and fixation in secondary IOL implantation after intracapsular extraction. *Int Ophthalmol.* 1986;9:151-160.
22. Banaee T, Sagheb S. Scleral fixation of intraocular lens in eyes with history of open globe injury. *J Pediatr Ophthalmol Strabismus.* 2011;48:292-297. doi:10.3928/01913913-20100818-01
23. Mahapatra SK, Rao NG. Visual outcome of pars plana vitrectomy with intraocular foreign body removal through sclerocorneal tunnel and sulcus-fixated intraocular lens implantation as a single procedure, in cases of metallic intraocular foreign body with traumatic cataract. *Indian J Ophthalmol.* 2010;58:115-118. doi:10.4103/0301-4738.60077
24. Zheng D, Wan P, Liang J, Song T, Liu Y. Comparison of clinical outcomes between iris fixated anterior chamber intraocular lenses and scleral fixated posterior chamber intraocular lenses in Marfan's syndrome with lens subluxation. *Clin Experiment Ophthalmol.* 2011;40(3):268-274. doi:10.1111/j.1442-9071.2011.02612.x
25. Kwong YY, Yuen HK, Lam RF, Lee VY, Rao SK, Lam DS. Comparison of outcomes of primary scleral-fixated versus primary anterior chamber intraocular lens implantation in complicated cataract surgeries. *Ophthalmology.* 2007;114:80-85. doi:10.1016/j.ophtha.2005.11.024
26. Olsen TW, Pribila JT. Pars plana vitrectomy with endoscope-guided sutured posterior chamber intraocular lens implantation in children and adults. *Am J Ophthalmol.* 2011;151:287-296. doi:10.1016/j.ajo.2010.08.026
27. Sharkey JA, Murray TG. Identification of the ora serrata and ciliary body by transillumination in eyes undergoing transscleral fixation of posterior chamber intraocular lenses. *Ophthalmic Surg.* 1994;25:479-480.

28. Pavlin CJ, Rootman D, Arshinoff S, Harasiewicz K, Foster FS. Determination of haptic position of transsclerally fixated posterior chamber intraocular lenses by ultrasound biomicroscopy. *J Cataract Refract Surg.* 1993;19:573-577.

29. Zhang ZD, Shen LJ, Liu XQ, Chen YQ, Qu J. Injection and suturing technique for scleral fixation foldable lens in the vitrectomized eye. *Retina.* 2010;30:353-356. doi:10.1097/IAE.0b013e3181c7021d

30. Kim DH, Heo JW, Hwang SW, Lee JH, Chung H. Modified transscleral fixation using combined temporary haptic externalization and injector intraocular lens implantation. *J Cataract Refract Surg.* 2010;36:707-711. doi:10.1016/j.jcrs.2009.11.030

31. Almashad GY, Abdelrahman AM, Khattab HA, Samir A. Four-point scleral fixation of posterior chamber intraocular lenses without scleral flaps. *Br J Ophthalmol.* 2010;94:693-695. doi:10.1136/bjo.2009.161349

32. Lin CP, Tseng HY. Suture fixation technique for posterior chamber intraocular lenses. *J Cataract Refract Surg.* 2004;30:1401-1404. doi:10.1016/j.jcrs.2003.11.044

33. Hoffman RS, Fine IH, Packer M. Scleral fixation without conjunctival dissection. *J Cataract Refract Surg.* 2006;32:1907-1912. doi:10.1016/j.jcrs.2006.05.029

34. Hoffman RS, Fine IH, Packer M, Rozenberg I. Scleral fixation using suture retrieval through a scleral tunnel. *J Cataract Refract Surg.* 2006;32:1259-1263. doi:10.1016/j.jcrs.2006.02.065

35. Caca I, Sahin A, Ari S, Alakus F. Posterior chamber lens implantation with scleral fixation in children with traumatic cataract. *J Pediatr Ophthalmol Strabismus.* 2011;48:226-231. doi:10.3928/01913913-20100719-01

36. Ma KT, Kang SY, Shin JY, Kim NR, Seong GJ, Kim CY. Modified Siepser sliding knot technique for scleral fixation of subluxated posterior chamber intraocular lens. *J Cataract Refract Surg.* 2010;36:6-8. doi:10.1016/j.jcrs.2009.07.048

37. Oetting TA, Tsui JY, Szeto AT. Sliding internal knot technique for late in-the-bag intraocular lens decentration. *J Cataract Refract Surg.* 2011;37:810-813. doi:10.1016/j.jcrs.2011.03.018

38. Bas AM, Bulacio JL, Carrizo R. Monoscleral fixation for posterior chamber intraocular lenses in cases of posterior capsule rupture. *Ann Ophthalmol.* 1990;22:341-345.

39. Lorente R, de Rojas V, Vazquez de Parga P, et al. Management of late spontaneous in-the-bag intraocular lens dislocation: Retrospective analysis of 45 cases. *J Cataract Refract Surg.* 2010;36:1270-1282. doi:10.1016/j.jcrs.2010.01.035

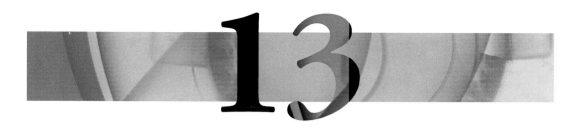

Glued Intraocular Lens

Glued Intrascleral Haptic Fixation
of a Posterior Chamber Intraocular Lens

Ashvin Agarwal, MS and Amar Agarwal, MS, FRCS, FRCOphth

Posterior capsular rupture can occur in the early learning curve of phacoemulsification.[1-15] The fibrin glue-assisted (Figure 13-1) sutureless intraocular lens (IOL) implantation with scleral tuck (glued IOL technique), introduced by Dr. Amar Agarwal can be used in eyes with inadequate anterior capsular rim and deficient posterior capsule.[3-7] The scleral tuck and intrascleral haptic fixation of a posterior chamber IOL was first introduced by Gabor and Pavilidis.[8] Maggi and Maggi[9] had previously performed a sutureless scleral fixation of a special IOL.

PREPARING THE EYE

The corneal white-to-white (WTW) diameter is measured. If the horizontal WTW diameter is approximately 11 mm, a horizontal glued IOL with scleral flaps at the 3- and 9-o'clock positions is implanted. As suggested by Dr. Jeevan Ladi,[16] if the WTW diameter is more than 11 mm, a vertical glued IOL is preferred where the scleral flaps are made at the 12- and 6-o'clock positions to allow exteriorization of a greater length of the haptic (Figure 13-2). To begin, scleral flaps 2.5 mm × 2.5 mm in size are marked 180 degrees apart (Figure 13-3). A scleral marker (Epsilon, Irving, TX), designed by Dr. Ashvin Agarwal, is used to place marks on the sclera 180 degrees apart and the scleral flaps are created (Figures 13-4 and 13-5). This special marker also marks the scleral flap areas. Any bleeding vessels are cauterized. A sutureless 23- to 25-gauge trocar cannula (Figure 13-6) is used for infusion. It should be verified that the tip of the infusion cannula is in the vitreous cavity before starting the infusion. For miotic pupils, an iris retractor is used to retract the iris and to verify the position of the infusion cannula. Alternatively, an anterior chamber maintainer may also be fixed parallel to the iris and away from the pupillary axis (Figure 13-7). An anterior chamber maintainer has the advantage of being easily available and reusable. The disadvantage is that inflow from the anterior chamber maintainer pushes the iris backward, thus increasing the risk of hitting the iris root while creating the sclerotomy. To avoid this, infusion

Agarwal A.
*Posterior Capsular Rupture: A Practical Guide
to Prevention and Management* (pp 127-154).
© 2014 Taylor & Francis Group.

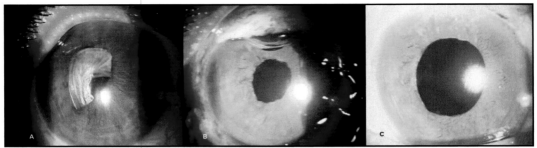

Figure 13-1. Subluxated IOL explanted and replaced by a glued IOL. (A) Preoperative slit lamp image showing an anterior subluxated IOL. (B) Postoperative day 1 of the glued IOL after the subluxated IOL was explanted. (C) Three months after surgery.

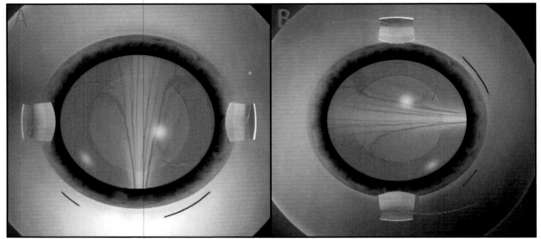

Figure 13-2. (A) Horizontal glued IOL. Note the amount of haptic available to tuck and glue is less. (B) Vertical glued IOL. Note the amount of haptic available to tuck and glue is much more.

flow of fluid should be temporarily stopped while creating the 20-gauge sclerotomies. Two straight sclerotomies with a 20-gauge needle are made approximately 1.0 mm from the limbus under the existing scleral flaps (Figure 13-8). The sclerotomies are directed obliquely into the mid-vitreous cavity to avoid hitting the iris root, which can occur if the sclerotomies are made in a horizontal direction. Vitrectomy is then performed using a 20-, 23-, or 25-gauge vitrectomy probe. A good vitrectomy is crucial so that no vitreous traction occurs and the chances of retinal breaks or retinal detachment decreases. Both 23- and 25-gauge vitrectomy probes can be passed through the sclerotomy under the scleral flap to remove anterior and mid-vitreous (Figure 13-9), whereas 20-gauge vitrectomy probes can be passed through the sideport.

INTRAOCULAR LENS TYPES

Glued IOL implantation can be performed with a rigid polymethyl methacrylate (PMMA) IOL, 3-piece posterior chamber IOL, or IOLs with modified PMMA haptics. Therefore, there is no need to have an entire inventory of special IOLs such as sutured scleral-fixated IOLs with eyelets or anterior chamber IOLs. The authors prefer the 3-piece IOL, as the haptics do not break compared to a single-piece nonfoldable IOL. A foldable, 3-piece IOL is even better, as the incision does not need

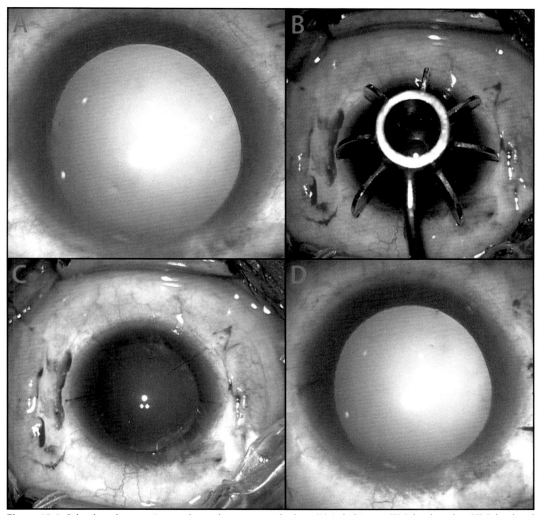

Figure 13-3. Scleral marker creating marks on the cornea and sclera. (A) Aphakic eye. (B) Scleral marker. (C) Scleral and corneal marks made. (D) Scleral flaps made.

to be enlarged. The length of a normal foldable, 3-piece IOL is 13 mm. The STAAR Surgical lens (STAAR AQ2010V; Monrovia, CA) is 13.5 mm in length, which allows a longer length of haptic to be externalized. The B-cartridge (Alcon, Fort Worth, TX) works perfectly with the AQ2010V and the Royale injector (Asico, Westmont, IL). The 3-piece, nonfoldable IOLs are also 13.5 mm in length. In the event of PMMA posterior chamber IOL or 3-piece IOL dislocation, the same IOL can be repositioned, thereby reducing the need for further manipulation. Single-piece, foldable IOLs cannot be used for the glued IOL technique.

GLUED INTRAOCULAR LENS HAPTIC EXTERIORIZATION

A plunger-type injector allows for better coordination of implantation, although a screw mechanism-type injector may also be used. With the latter, the assistant gently maneuvers the IOL forward as the surgeon holds the injector with one hand and the glued IOL forceps (Epsilon) with the other hand. While introducing the injector, it is advisable to have the injector tip within the

Figure 13-4. Dr. Ashvin Agarwal's scleral marker creates marks for the scleral flaps. The device measures 11 mm so the surgeon can know immediately whether the WTW diameter is too large.

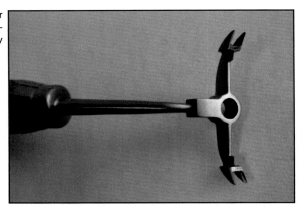

Figure 13-5. Scleral flap creation. (A) The knife first makes half-thickness marks. (B) The dissector passes through one end of the flap.

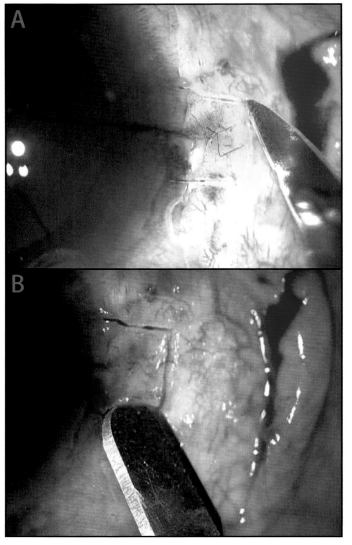

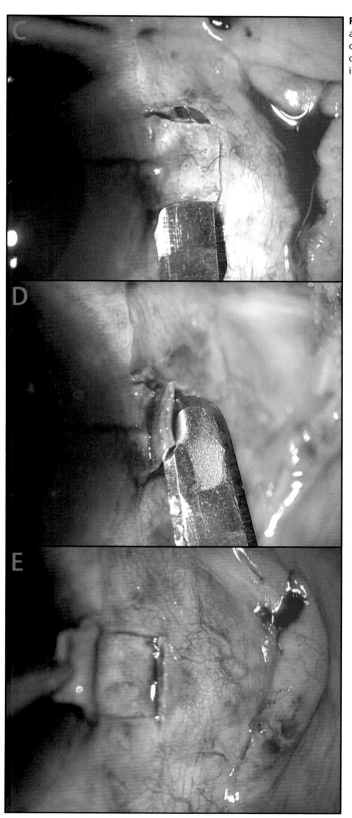

Figure 13-5 (continued). Scleral flap creation. (C) Dissector comes out from the other end. (D) The dissector is moved outward to complete the flap. (E) The flap is lifted and checked.

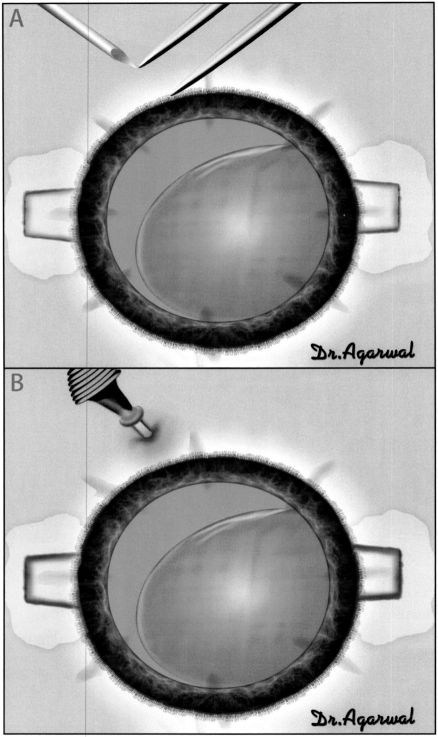

Figure 13-6. Insertion of 23-gauge trocar and cannula for glued IOL implantation surgery. (A) A 23-gauge trocar is placed 3.0 mm from the limbus. The distance is measured using a caliper. (B) The trocar is inserted into the pars plana.

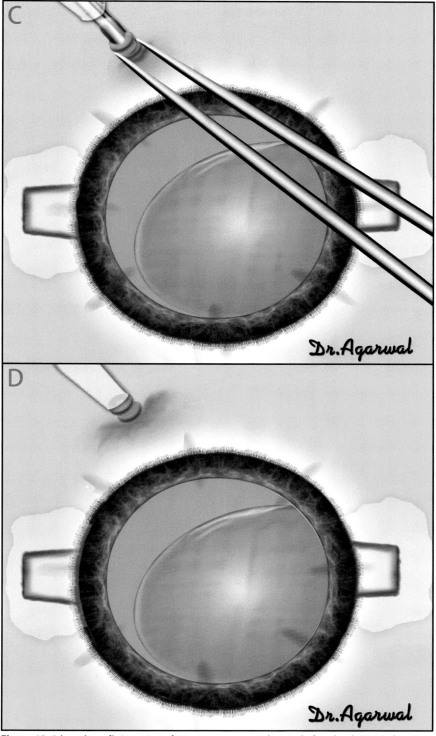

Figure 13-6 (continued). Insertion of 23-gauge trocar and cannula for glued IOL implantation surgery. (C–D) The inserter is removed and an infusion cannula connected to the infusion bottle is inserted.

Figure 13-7. Anterior chamber maintainer.

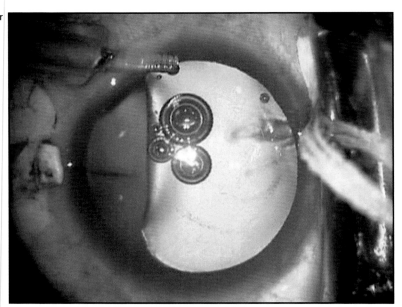

Figure 13-8. Sclerotomy is made 1 mm from the limbus under the scleral flap using a 20-gauge needle.

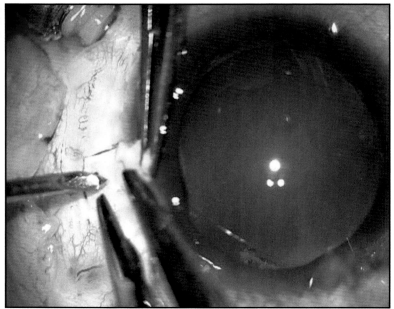

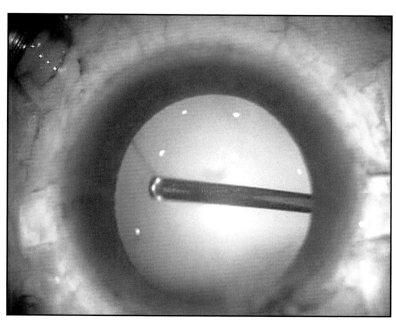

Figure 13-9. A 23-gauge vitrectomy probe is used to remove anterior and mid-vitreous.

mouth of the incision and not use wound-assisted injection of the IOL, which can lead to a sudden, uncontrolled entry of the IOL into the eye and a consequent IOL drop into the vitreous. After the 3-piece, foldable IOL is loaded (Figure 13-10), the haptic should be left slightly out of the cartridge (Figure 13-11). The tip of the leading haptic points to the left in the *lucky seven* sign, to use a term coined by Dr. Thomas Oetting.[17] The cartridge is passed into the anterior chamber (Figure 13-12). The glued IOL forceps are passed through the sclerotomy and grasp the tip of the haptic. The IOL is then gradually injected into the eye. If the injector is the screw-mechanism type, the assistant screws the injector. The haptic should not be externalized until the optic completely unfolds inside the eye to prevent breakage of the optic. After the optic is unfolded fully, the glued IOL forceps pull the haptic and externalize it. At the same time, the cartridge is brought out of the eye and the second haptic is allowed to trail out of the eye. This is in the shape of an upright "C."[17] The haptic is then transferred to an assistant.

The trailing haptic is then caught with the first glued IOL forceps and flexed into the anterior chamber (Figure 13-13). The haptic is transferred from the first forceps to the second forceps using the handshake technique (Figure 13-14). The second forceps are passed through the sideport. The first forceps are then passed through the sclerotomy under the scleral flap. The haptic is transferred from the second forceps back to the first using the handshake technique again. The haptic tip is grasped with the first forceps and pulled toward the sclerotomy and externalized. If the haptic is below the iris, the surgeon should use the handshake technique (Figure 13-15).

No-Assistant Technique

Dr. George Beiko[18] has suggested placing silicone plugs from an iris hook onto the haptic that has been externalized, which prevents the haptic from slipping back (Figure 13-16). Dr. Priya Narang[19] has suggested a no-assistant technique whereby the trailing haptic is passed into the eye near the inferior portion so that (due to physic principles) the leading haptic cannot slip back.

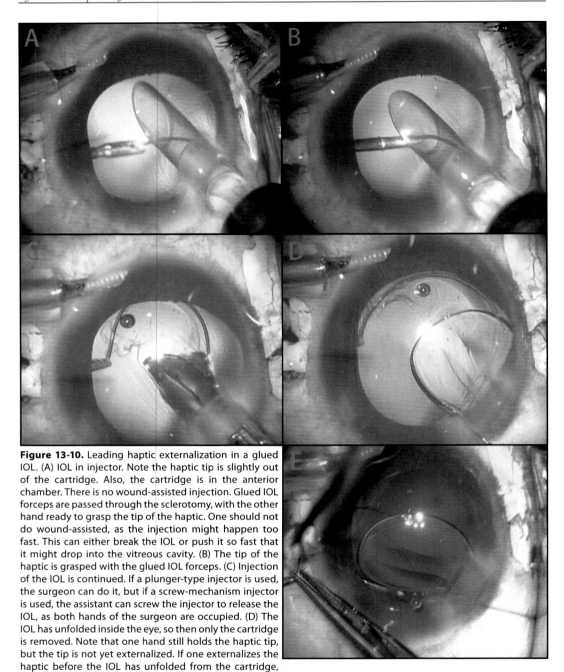

Figure 13-10. Leading haptic externalization in a glued IOL. (A) IOL in injector. Note the haptic tip is slightly out of the cartridge. Also, the cartridge is in the anterior chamber. There is no wound-assisted injection. Glued IOL forceps are passed through the sclerotomy, with the other hand ready to grasp the tip of the haptic. One should not do wound-assisted, as the injection might happen too fast. This can either break the IOL or push it so fast that it might drop into the vitreous cavity. (B) The tip of the haptic is grasped with the glued IOL forceps. (C) Injection of the IOL is continued. If a plunger-type injector is used, the surgeon can do it, but if a screw-mechanism injector is used, the assistant can screw the injector to release the IOL, as both hands of the surgeon are occupied. (D) The IOL has unfolded inside the eye, so then only the cartridge is removed. Note that one hand still holds the haptic tip, but the tip is not yet externalized. If one externalizes the haptic before the IOL has unfolded from the cartridge, the IOL can break. (E) The haptic is externalized, and the assistant tries to grasp the haptic so it does not fall back inside the eye. (Reprinted from Agarwal A, Jacob S, Kumar DA, Agarwal A, Narasimhan S, Agarwal A. Handshake technique for glued intrascleral haptic fixation of a posterior chamber intraocular lens. *J Cataract Refract Surg.* 2013;3:317-322, with permission from Elsevier.)

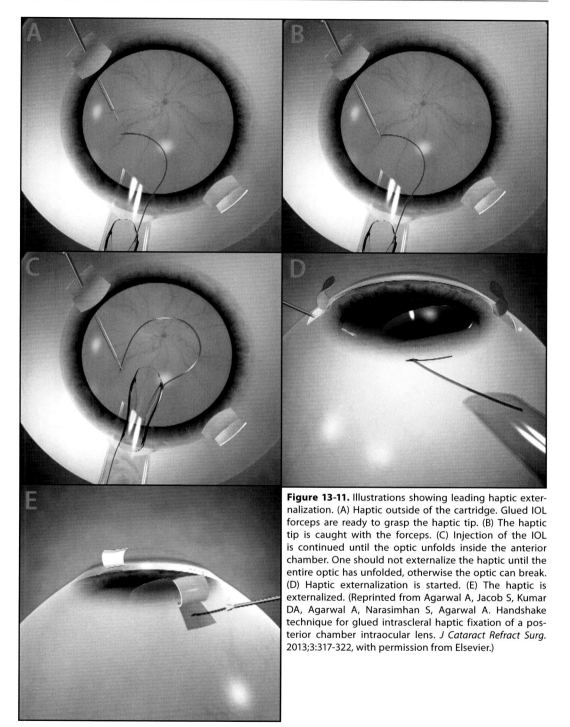

Figure 13-11. Illustrations showing leading haptic externalization. (A) Haptic outside of the cartridge. Glued IOL forceps are ready to grasp the haptic tip. (B) The haptic tip is caught with the forceps. (C) Injection of the IOL is continued until the optic unfolds inside the anterior chamber. One should not externalize the haptic until the entire optic has unfolded, otherwise the optic can break. (D) Haptic externalization is started. (E) The haptic is externalized. (Reprinted from Agarwal A, Jacob S, Kumar DA, Agarwal A, Narasimhan S, Agarwal A. Handshake technique for glued intrascleral haptic fixation of a posterior chamber intraocular lens. _J Cataract Refract Surg._ 2013;3:317-322, with permission from Elsevier.)

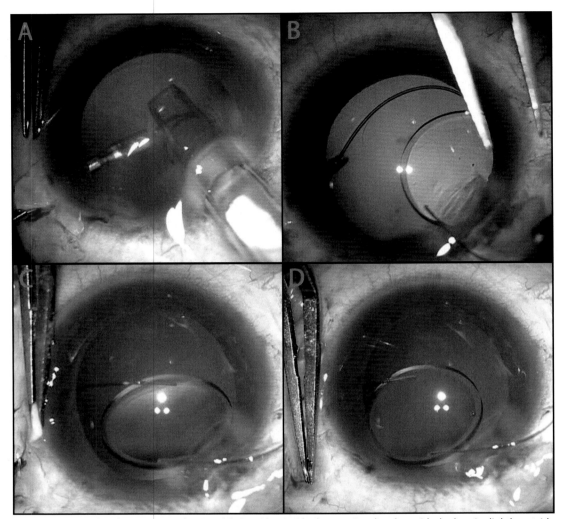

Figure 13-12. Leading haptic externalization. (A) Cartridge inside the anterior chamber with the haptic slightly outside (lucky seven sign). The glued IOL forceps are passed through the sclerotomy and is ready to grasp the haptic tip. (B) The haptic tip are grasped with the glued IOL forceps. Foldable IOL injection is continued with one hand. This injector has a pushing mechanism, so one hand can be used. If the injector has a screw mechanism, the assistant continues the injection. (C) The forceps pull the haptic while injection of the foldable IOL is continued. (D) The haptic is externalized. The assistant then holds the haptic. The trailing haptic lies outside the wound with an upright "C" sign.

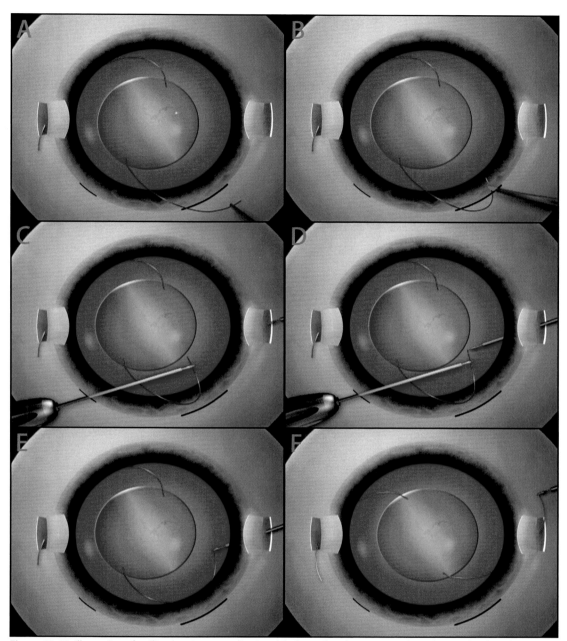

Figure 13-13. Illustration of trailing haptic externalization. (A) The trailing haptic is caught with one glued IOL forceps. (B) The haptic is flexed into the anterior chamber. (C) The haptic is transferred from the first forceps to the second forceps using the handshake technique. The second forceps are passed through the sideport. (D) The first forceps are passed through the sclerotomy under the scleral flap. (E) The haptic is then transferred from the second forceps back to the first using the handshake technique. The haptic tip is grasped with the first forceps. (F) The haptic is pulled toward the sclerotomy and externalized. (Reprinted from Agarwal A, Jacob S, Kumar DA, Agarwal A, Narasimhan S, Agarwal A. Handshake technique for glued intrascleral haptic fixation of a posterior chamber intraocular lens. _J Cataract Refract Surg._ 2013;3:317-322, with permission from Elsevier.)

Figure 13-14. Handshake technique for trailing haptic. (A) Glued IOL forceps are passed through the sideport. (B) The trailing haptic is grasped with forceps and flexed to make it enter the anterior chamber. (C) Trailing haptic is passed into the anterior chamber and the haptic grasp is shifted from one forceps to the other using the handshake technique. Note the dimpling on the cornea as the main incision is opened due to the forceps passage. (Reprinted from Agarwal A, Jacob S, Kumar DA, Agarwal A, Narasimhan S, Agarwal A. Handshake technique for glued intrascleral haptic fixation of a posterior chamber intraocular lens. *J Cataract Refract Surg.* 2013;3:317-322, with permission from Elsevier.)

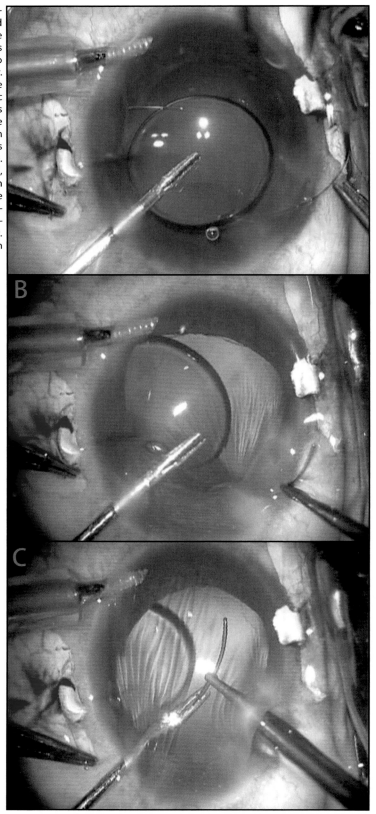

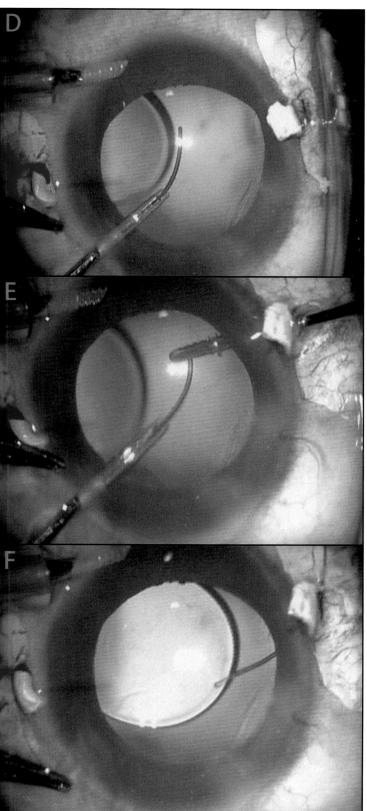

Figure 13-14 (continued). Handshake technique for trailing haptic. (D) The trailing haptic is caught with forceps and passed through the sideport. Note that there is no dimpling on the cornea as the main incision is closed. It is now easy to see the tip of the haptic. (E) The glued IOL forceps are passed through the sclerotomy and the tip of the haptic is grasped. Once again, the handshake technique helps pass the haptic from one forceps to the other. (F) The trailing haptic is externalized. (Reprinted from Agarwal A, Jacob S, Kumar DA, Agarwal A, Narasimhan S, Agarwal A. Handshake technique for glued intrascleral haptic fixation of a posterior chamber intraocular lens. *J Cataract Refract Surg.* 2013;3:317-322, with permission from Elsevier.)

Figure 13-15. Handshake technique. (A) The foldable IOL haptic is below the iris. (B) One forceps with the end opened are passed through the opposite sclerotomy site while other forceps are ready to receive the haptic. (C) The trailing haptic is passed into the anterior chamber using the handshake technique, and the haptic grasp is shifted from one forceps to another. (Reprinted from Agarwal A, Jacob S, Kumar DA, Agarwal A, Narasimhan S, Agarwal A. Handshake technique for glued intrascleral haptic fixation of a posterior chamber intraocular lens. *J Cataract Refract Surg.* 2013;3:317-322, with permission from Elsevier.)

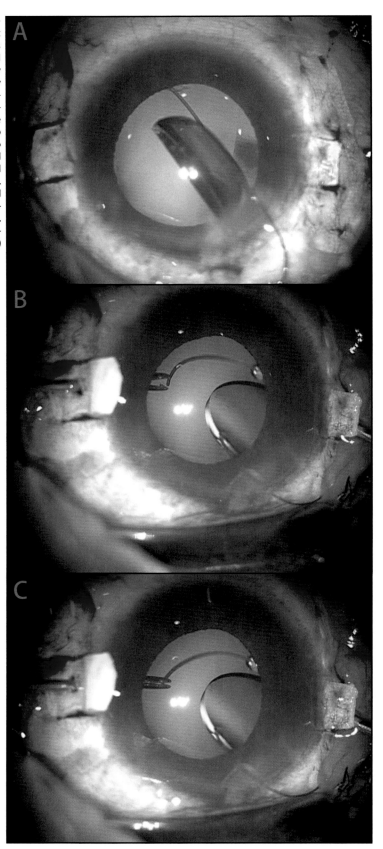

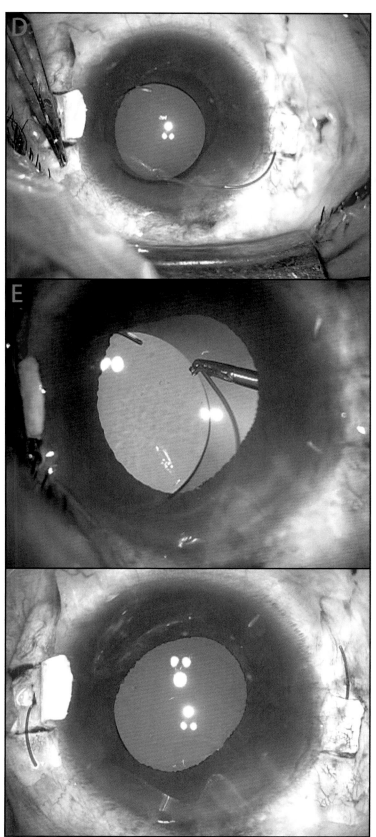

Figure 13-15 (continued).
Handshake technique. (D) One haptic is externalized and an assistant holds the haptic. (E) The trailing haptic is caught with the end-open forceps. (F) Both haptics are externalized under the scleral flaps. (Reprinted from Agarwal A, Jacob S, Kumar DA, Agarwal A, Narasimhan S, Agarwal A. Handshake technique for glued intrascleral haptic fixation of a posterior chamber intraocular lens. _J Cataract Refract Surg._ 2013;3:317-322, with permission from Elsevier.)

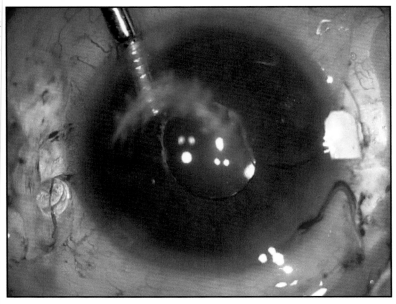

Figure 13-16. Beiko's modification. Silicone tire of iris hook prevents the haptic from slipping back into the vitreous cavity.

Holding the tip of the haptic with forceps with one hand while injecting the IOL with the other decreases the chances of the IOL dropping into the vitreous cavity because of the following:

- The tip of the haptic is caught with the forceps.
- The trailing haptic is still outside the eye. If the forceps accidentally release the leading haptic, the trailing haptic can still be caught, and the IOL would not fall into the vitreous cavity.

The IOL position is then assessed. The IOL should be stable without being held by any instrument. If the haptic starts slipping back through the sclerotomy, then it is possible that the following occurred:

- The eye is large and has a large WTW diameter (in which case a vertical glued IOL would have to be done).
- The sclerotomy made is too far back (so very little haptic has been externalized).

If the haptics are slipping back, a fresh sclerotomy should be made more anterior to the previous one. The haptic should be pushed back into the vitreous cavity and, using the handshake technique, the haptic should again be grasped and re-externalized through the fresh anterior sclerotomy. Once again, IOL stability should be assessed. Vitrectomy is then performed around the sclerotomy.

SCHARIOTH SCLERAL POCKET AND INTRASCLERAL HAPTIC TUCK

Dr. Gabor Scharioth performed the first intrascleral haptic fixation in 2006.[8] It is the intrascleral haptic fixation that gives stability to the IOL. A bent, 26-gauge needle (Figure 13-17) is used to create a scleral tunnel at the edge of the flap where the haptic is externalized (Figure 13-18). The haptic is then flexed and tucked into the scleral pocket. This Scharioth scleral pocket can be created even before the eye is opened. The 26-gauge needle is marked with the marker pen to leave a mark in the sclera where the scleral pocket is created (Figure 13-19). A blunt rod can be used to

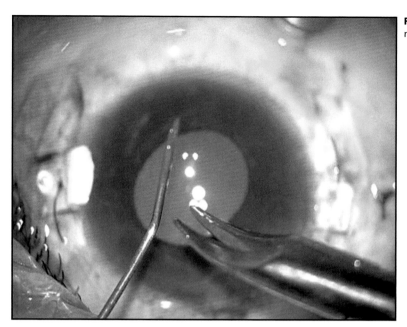

Figure 13-17. A 26-gauge needle is bent like a keratome.

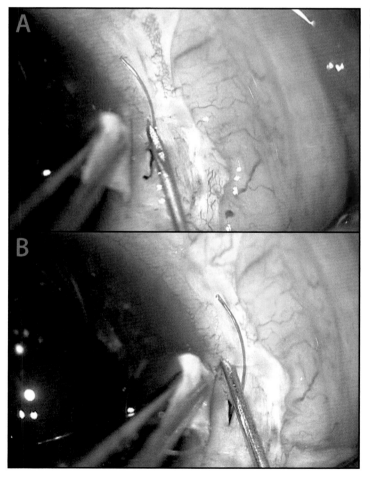

Figure 13-18. Scharioth scleral pocket creation with intrascleral haptic tuck. (A) A 26-gauge needle creates a scleral tunnel at the edge of the flap where the haptic is externalized. (B) Scharioth scleral pocket.

Figure 13-18 (continued). Scharioth scleral pocket creation with intrascleral haptic tuck. (C) The haptic is flexed to be tucked into the scleral pocket. (D) The haptic is tucked in the scleral pocket. (E) The IOL is centered and stable with the haptics tucked.

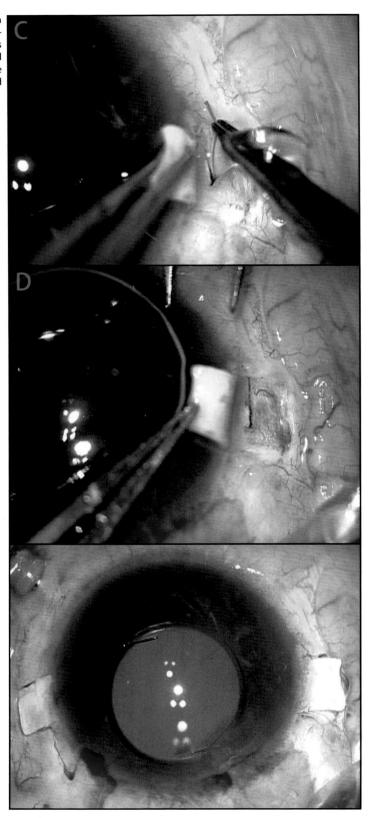

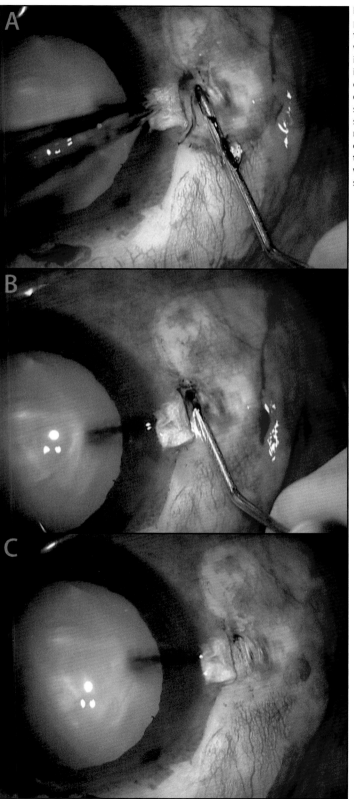

Figure 13-19. Marked Scharioth scleral pocket creation before IOL implantation. (A) A 26-gauge needle is inked with the marker pen to leave a mark in the sclera where the scleral pocket is created. This can be done before opening the eye, as it will have to be done adjacent to the area where the sclerotomy will be made. (B) Marked scleral pocket created by 26-gauge needle. (C) Marked scleral pocket is created. It is now easy to know where the scleral pocket is located. Another way is to pass a rod in the area of the sclera pocket to check its location.

Figure 13-20. Air bubble in the anterior chamber.

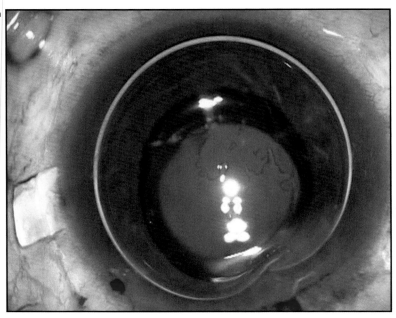

open up the tunnel if difficulty is experienced during tucking. Air is then injected into the anterior chamber, and the infusion cannula is turned off (Figure 13-20).

FIBRIN GLUE

The authors use the fibrin glue kit Reliseal (Reliance Life Science, Thane, Maharashtra, India) or Tisseel (Baxter, Deerfield, IL). Commercially available fibrin glue is virus inactivated and is checked for viral antigen and antibodies with polymerase chain reaction; thus, the chances of infection transmission are very low. The glue is applied under the flaps, and it can also be used to seal the conjunctival and clear corneal incisions (Figure 13-21).

The following shows the multifactorial roles of fibrin glue in glued IOL surgery:

- The glue helps to seal the haptic to the sclera, which gives extra support to the intrascleral haptic tuck in the early postoperative period. Surgical fibrosis occurs once the glue has degraded.

- The glue, in the initial period and in the later surgical fibrosis, seals the flaps hermetically, thus avoiding ingress or egress of fluid through the sclerotomies. This prevents endophthalmitis, even years later.

- The glue prevents any trabeculectomy opening, as the flaps are now firmly stuck.

- The glue helps to seal the conjunctiva, as well as the clear corneal incisions.

After removing the speculum, the globe is again checked for hypotony. If soft hypotony is found, balanced salt solution is injected into the anterior chamber until the globe is adequately firm again. It is advisable to leave a small air bubble in the anterior chamber.

Postoperatively, the patients should be closely monitored, as their cases are generally complicated (Figure 13-22). Postoperative antibiotic steroids are given for 6 weeks. In case of anterior chamber reaction, subconjunctival antibiotic steroids can also be prescribed. If a temporary elevation of intraocular pressure occurs, antiglaucoma medications can also be prescribed.

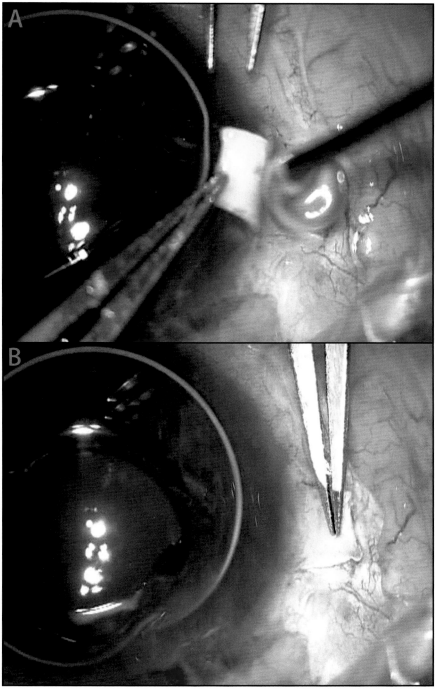

Figure 13-21. Fibrin glue application. (A) Fibrin glue is applied under the flaps. (B) Scleral flaps are stuck.

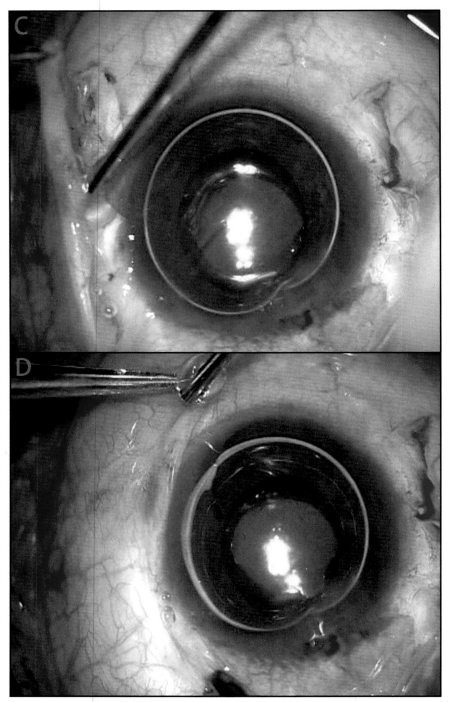

Figure 13-21 (continued). Fibrin glue application. (C) Fibrin glue is applied to seal the conjunctiva. (D) Conjunctiva is sealed with the glue.

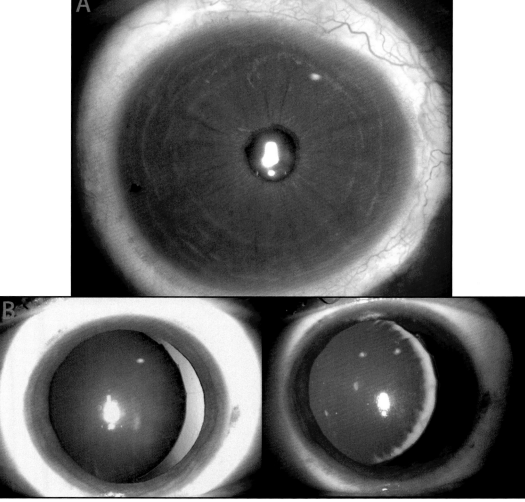

Figure 13-22. Glued IOL. (A) Glued IOL in the right eye 1.5 years postoperatively. (B) Subluxated cataract in the left eye.

STABILITY OF THE INTRAOCULAR LENS HAPTIC

Numerous animal studies have shown that fibrin glue is still present at 4 to 6 weeks postoperatively. Because postoperative fibrosis starts early, the flaps can become stuck secondary to fibrosis, even prior to full degradation of the glue. The ensuing fibrosis acts to form a firm scaffold around the haptic, which prevents movement along the long axis (Figure 13-23A). To further make the IOL stable, the authors tuck the haptic tip into the scleral wall through the tunnel. This prevents all movement of the haptic along the transverse axis as well (Figure 13-23B). The stability of the lens is first ensured by tucking the haptics into the scleral pocket created. The tissue glue then provides extra stability and it also seals the flap down. Externalization of the greater part of the haptics along its curvature stabilizes the axial positioning of the IOL, thereby preventing any IOL tilt.

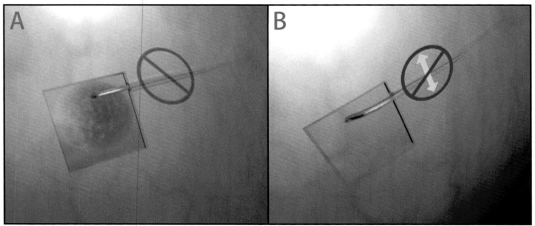

Figure 13-23. Stability of the IOL. (A) Long axis movement is prevented by the tissue glue initially and later by sub flap fibrosis. (B) Transverse axis movement is prevented by the scleral tuck.

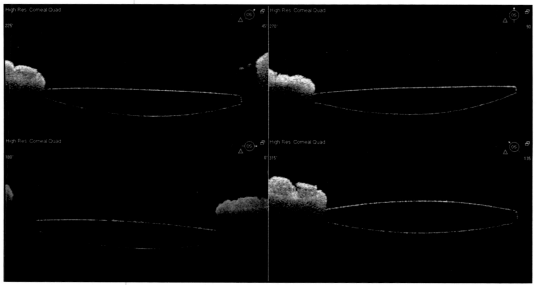

Figure 13-24. Anterior segment optical coherence tomography (OCT) showing 360 degrees of good centration of the IOL.

ADVANTAGES OF GLUED INTRAOCULAR LENSES

The following list shows the advantages of performing glued intrascleral haptic fixation of posterior chamber IOLs:

- No special IOLs are required.

- Tilt is avoided easily if the limbus-sclerotomy distance is kept equal on both sides (see Figures 13-13 to 13-24).

- Less pseudophakodonesis occurs because the IOL haptic is stuck beneath the flap and into the tunnel which prevents movement of the haptic, thus reducing pseudophakodonesis.

- Less uveitis-glaucoma-hyphema (UGH) syndrome occurs. We expect less incidence of UGH syndrome in fibrin glue-assisted IOL implantation compared with sutured scleral-fixated IOL

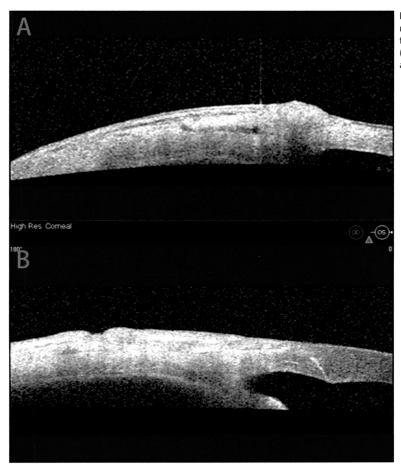

Figure 13-25. (A) Anterior segment OCT showing the scleral flap placement on day 1 and (B) adhesion well maintained at 6 weeks.

implantation. This is because in the former, the IOL is well stabilized and stuck onto the scleral bed, thereby having decreased intraocular mobility, whereas in the latter, there is the increased possibility of IOL movement or persistent rub over the ciliary body.

- Late subluxation due to suture-related complications such as suture erosion, suture knot exposure, or dislocation of the IOL after suture disintegration or broken suture, are avoided.

- Rapidity and ease of surgery are seen. The time taken for passing the suture into the IOL haptic eyelets in a scleral-fixated IOL to ensure good centering before tying down the knots and time spent suturing the scleral flaps and closing the conjunctiva is significantly reduced. The risk of retinal photic injury would also be reduced with this technique due to the short surgical time.

- The use of fibrin glue has been shown to provide airtight closure. By the time the fibrin glue starts to degrade, surgical adhesions would have already occurred in the scleral bed. This is well established in follow-up anterior segment OCT (Figure 13-25), where perfect scleral flap adhesion is observed postoperatively.

- Implantation of a multifocal glued IOL. In the event of a posterior capsular rupture, it is not advisable to place a multifocal IOL in the sulcus due to the possibility of postoperative decentration. If in-the-bag multifocal IOL implantation is not possible, implantation of a glued multifocal IOL may be preferred as the IOL is stable with no postoperative decentration of the IOL occurring from its intraoperative positioning.

CONCLUSION

Glued IOL implantation can help patients with posterior capsular rupture. The biggest advantages are the speed of surgery, a less traumatic surgery, and that pseudophakodonesis of the IOL does not occur.

REFERENCES

1. Vajpayee RB, Sharma N, Dada T, et al. Management of posterior capsule tears. *Surv Ophthal.* 2001;45:473-488.
2. Wu MC, Bhandari A. Managing the broken capsule. *Curr Opin Ophthalmol.* 2008;19:36-40.
3. Agarwal A, Kumar DA, Jacob S, et al. Fibrin glue–assisted sutureless posterior chamber intraocular lens implantation in eyes with deficient posterior capsules. *J Cataract Refract Surg.* 2008;34:1433-1438.
4. Prakash G, Kumar DA, Jacob S, et al. Anterior segment optical coherence tomography–aided diagnosis and primary posterior chamber intraocular lens implantation with fibrin glue in traumatic phacocele with scleral perforation. *J Cataract Refract Surg.* 2009;35:782-784.
5. Prakash G, Jacob S, Kumar DA, et al. Femtosecond assisted keratoplasty with fibrin glue–assisted sutureless posterior chamber lens implantation: a new triple procedure. *J Cataract Refract Surg.* 2009;35(6):973-979.
6. Agarwal A, Kumar DA, Prakash G, et al. Fibrin glue–assisted sutureless posterior chamber intraocular lens implantation in eyes with deficient posterior capsules [reply to letter]. *J Cataract Refract Surg.* 2009;35:795-796.
7. Nair V, Kumar DA, Prakash G, et al. Bilateral spontaneous in-the-bag anterior subluxation of PC IOL managed with glued IOL technique: a case report. *Eye Contact Lens.* 2009;35(4):215-217.
8. Gabor SGB, Pavilidis MM. Sutureless intrascleral posterior chamber intraocular lens fixation. *J Cataract Refract Surg.* 2007;33:1851-1854.
9. Maggi R, Maggi C. Sutureless scleral fixation of intraocular lenses. *J Cataract Refract Surg.* 1997;23:1289-1294.
10. Teichmann KD, Teichmann IAM. The torque and tilt gamble. *J Cataract Refract Surg.* 1997;23:413-418.
11. Jacobi KW, Jagger WS. Physical forces involved in pseudophacodonesis and iridodonesis. *Albrecht Von Graefes Arch Klin Exp Ophthalmol.* 1981;216:49-53.
12. Price MO, Price FW Jr, Werner L, et al. Late dislocation of scleral-sutured posterior chamber intraocular lenses. *J Cataract Refract Surg.* 2005;31(7):1320-1326.
13. Solomon K, Gussler JR, Gussler C, Van Meter WS. Incidence and management of complications of transsclerally sutured posterior chamber lenses. *J Cataract Refract Surg.* 1993;19:488-493.
14. Asadi R, Kheirkhah A. Long-term results of scleral fixation of posterior chamber intraocular lenses in children. *Ophthalmology.* 2008;115(1):67-72.
15. Lanzetta P, Menchini U, Virgili G, et al. Scleral fixated intraocular lenses: an angiographic study. *Retina.* 1998;18:515-520.
16. Ladi JS, Shah NA. Vertical fixation with fibrin glue-assisted secondary posterior chamber intraocular lens implantation in a case of surgical aphakia. *Indian J Ophthalmol.* 2013;61(3):126-129.
17. Agarwal A, Agarwal A, Jacob S, et al. Comprehending IOL signs and the significance in Glued IOL surgery. *J Refract Surg.* 2013;29(2):79.
18. Beiko G, Steinert R. Modification of externalized haptic support of glued intraocular lens technique. *J Cataract Refract Surg.* 2013;39(3):323-325. doi: 10.1016/j.jcrs.2013.01.017.
19. Narang P. Modified method of haptic externalization of posterior chamber intraocular lens in fibrin glue-assisted intrascleral fixation: no-assistant technique. *J Cataract Refract Surg.* 2013;39:4-7.

IV

Special Cases and Complications of Posterior Capsular Rupture

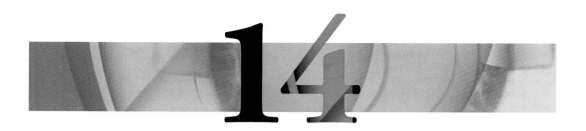

Femtosecond Laser Refractive Cataract Surgery and Posterior Capsular Rupture

Zoltán Z. Nagy, MD, PhD, FEBO, DSc and
Michael Lawless, MBBS, FRANZCO, FRACS

The principles of phacoemulsification for cataract surgery have not changed much during the past 20 years. It has been and still is a manual procedure and the outcome is highly dependent on the surgeon's skill. Occasionally, even the most experienced and skilled surgeons may encounter difficulty with the posterior capsule, and possible further inconsistent surgical maneuvers can lead to cascading effects that may cause posterior capsular rupture. The recently developed femtosecond laser for refractive cataract surgery provides computer-controlled, precision laser surgery (Figure 14-1). Proper pharmacological dilation is very important before surgery[1] in case adhered-pupil mechanical dilation may be necessary with iris hook, Malyugin ring (MicroSurgical Technology, Redmond, WA), or with other types of mechanical dilators.

POSTERIOR CAPSULAR RUPTURE

The preservation of the posterior capsule during cataract surgery is of utmost importance to avoid possible complications such as loss of lens material into the vitreous, chronic inflammation, secondary glaucoma, cystoid macular edema, posterior chamber lens dislocation and subsequent monocular diplopia, unfavorable change in refraction and in higher order aberrations, and possible retinal detachment. The rate of posterior capsular damage is reported to be between 0.05% to 2.0%.[1,2] Signs of damaged posterior capsule are sudden deepening and fluctuations of the anterior chamber, pupillary dilatation at the moment the posterior capsule was torn, and the nucleus not being held by the phaco tip but rather jumping away.[1] Posterior capsular rupture can occur not only during phacoemulsification and irrigation/aspiration (I/A) of the cortex but also during hydrodissection.[2] A small tear in the anterior capsule, a small capsulorrhexis, or overzealous hydrodissection may result in rupture of the posterior capsule. Posterior polar cataract due to strong adherence to the posterior capsule may render cataract surgery also more

Agarwal A.
Posterior Capsular Rupture: A Practical Guide
to Prevention and Management (pp 157-163).
© 2014 Taylor & Francis Group.

Figure 14-1. The LenSx femtosecond laser. (Reprinted with permission from Alcon Laboratories, Fort Worth, TX.)

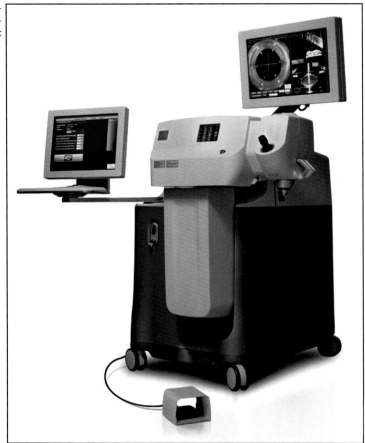

difficult to avoid capsular tears.[3] Other contributing factors are dense nucleus,[4] pseudoexfoliation, black or intumescent white cataracts, small pupil, history of blunt eye trauma, high myopia, high hyperopia, poor visibility for the surgeon (high brow, fluid pooling in the interpalpebral fissure due to abnormal head position, or draping problems with deep-set orbits), or anterior segment pathology that may cause poor visibility, such as band keratopathy, corneal scars, and pterygiums reaching the optical center. Human factors—such as an inexperienced surgeon, disoriented or anxious patients, and technical problems (eg, phacoemulsifier malfunction)—might be causative factors in posterior capsular damage.

INCIDENCE OF POSTERIOR CAPSULAR RUPTURE

Marques et al[5] reviewed 2646 eyes during phacoemulsification. The incidence of anterior tear was 0.8%, 40% of which extended into the posterior capsule and 20% of these eyes required vitrectomy. Unal et al[6] reviewed the medical residents' experience during phacoemulsification performed under topical anesthesia. It is worth noting that 5.3% of the cases had an anterior tear, the anterior capsulorrhexis was irregular in 9.3% of cases, and posterior capsular tear with vitreous loss occurred in 6.6% of the cases. Therefore, the level of surgical experience is an important factor in avoiding posterior capsular tear.[6]

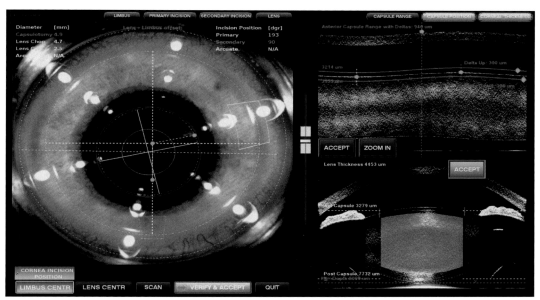

Figure 14-2. The proprietary inbuilt-optical coherence tomography (OCT) of the Alcon LenSx femtosecond laser identifies the anterior and posterior capsule and measures the density of the crystalline lens. The surgeon plans the femtosecond laser procedure based on the OCT results. Safety distance from the posterior capsule should be at least 500 μm. (Reprinted with permission from Alcon Laboratories, Fort Worth, TX.)

FEMTOSECOND CATARACT SURGERY

The clinical applications of the femtosecond laser in cataract refractive surgery are important to liquefy or fragment the lens, to create a well-centered and well-sized capsulotomy, to create all required corneal incisions with perfect dimensions and architecture, and to convert a manual, multitool, multistep procedure to one of laser-created, but surgeon-controlled, precision.[7,8]

To begin the femtosecond laser-assisted cataract surgery, a proprietary, curved patient interface is placed on the eye and the laser is lowered into the docking position. The LenSx femtosecond laser performs a proprietary 3-dimensional imaging that utilizes integrated real-time optical coherence tomography (OCT) technology to capture the entire anterior segment with one scan, projecting the detailed images of the ocular structures onto the video microscope screen in their true orientation. While taking the OCT measurements, the anterior and posterior capsules are identified and the density of the nucleus is also shown (Figures 14-2 and 14-3). At this point, the surgeon verifies the surgical plan and safety distance from the posterior and anterior capsules. The safety distance from the posterior capsule should be approximately 500 μm. The new software of the LenSx femtosecond laser is able to compensate for docking tilt.

Once the software calculates the laser treatment from the preprogrammed surgical parameters and patient data, the images of the proposed lens treatment pattern, anterior capsulotomy, and all corneal incisions are overlaid. The surgeon uses the touch keypad to modify centration and the placement of all incisions and confirms the proposed laser treatment as imaged on the screen. The surgeon then initiates the procedure with a press of the foot pedal. The entire procedure is displayed on the video screen and is completed in approximately 40 seconds. After having completed the femtosecond laser procedure, the patient is transferred to the main operating room.

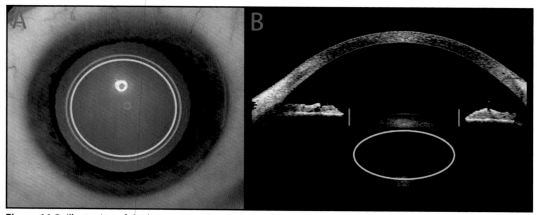

Figure 14-3. Illustration of the laser cuts within the eye superimposed on the (A) operating microscope and (B) OCT images. The yellow line represents the intended cut in the lens. The blue line shows the capsulotomy (centration and diameter) with the red line showing the corneal cuts.

Figure 14-4. Residual gas bubble within the dislocated crystalline lens after femtosecond laser cataract surgery. (Reprinted with permission from Michael Lawless, MBBS, FRANZCO, FRACS.)

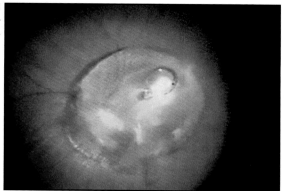

AVOIDING POSTERIOR CAPSULAR RUPTURE

During surgery, there are some special points to consider in order to avoid possible posterior capsular damage. As a first step, the surgeon identifies the paracentesis wound and opens it with a blunt spatula. Thereafter, the anterior chamber is filled with viscoelastic material. The primary corneal wound can be opened next. The capsule incision should be inspected meticulously and the surgeon should identify any areas of possible adhesions. The completely cut area of the capsule should be looked for and identified and possibly lifted with a rhexis needle (cystotome) or rhexis forceps. The contour of the femtosecond laser cut should be meticulously followed, and the round-shaped anterior capsule can be removed by this route. Pulling the capsule out with abrupt hand movements can cause anterior capsular tears, which might lead to anterior and posterior capsular damage. After removing the capsule, a slow hydrodissection should be performed. It should be carried out slowly and softly because a gas bubble may be present within the crystalline lens after fragmentation. With slow hydrodissection, the gas exits through the anterior capsule without a problem. With abrupt hydrodissection, a capsular blockage syndrome may result in rupture of the posterior capsule. With this cautious technique, posterior capsular rupture can be avoided in 100% of cases. Recently, 2 cases of capsular blockage syndrome have been reported during femtosecond laser cataract surgery.[9] In both cases, the overzealous hydrodissection was the most important causative factor in capsular rupture. Both cases required vitrectomy to remove the lens particles from the posterior pole of the eye (Figure 14-4).

During normal femtosecond laser refractive cataract surgery after successful hydrodissection, the surgeon enters the eye with the phaco head and the chopper. It is advisable to grab the lens near the perpendicular fragmentation line with 300 mm Hg and to chop it into 2 pieces with the chopper. Later, turn the lens and repeat the procedure with the other fragmentation line. Having 4 quadrants of the nucleus, the pieces can be easily removed using minimal phacoemulsification energy and time; therefore, the cumulative dissipation energy (CDE) can be minimized. After nucleus removal, the cortex should be removed with I/A similar to manual phacoemulsification. With a more conservative lens fragmentation pattern distance from the posterior capsule, a larger epinucleus occasionally creates a bowl which can be removed with the epinucleus program of the phaco machine, or simply with the I/A.

Posterior chamber lens implantation is similar to routine surgical techniques. At the end of surgery, the wound should be checked. Most cases do not require hydration because the wound itself is self-sealing. If there is rupture or other surgical trauma, the eye might require hydration. According to the surgeon's preference, intracameral antibiotics might be used to avoid postoperative intraocular complications.

In a case of softer lenses after removal of the anterior capsule, hydrodissection is usually not required and the central nucleus can be easily aspirated by using only the I/A tip. Anterior chamber depth should be closely monitored and maintained during surgery, especially with high myopes (and sometimes hyperopes) to ensure safety. It is especially important in younger patients operated under topical anesthesia. These patients can be anxious and exert pressure against the speculum, consequently causing higher intraocular pressure (IOP).

INTRAOPERATIVE CAPSULAR BLOCK SYNDROME

Intraoperative capsular block syndrome (CBS) during routine phacoemulsification is an uncommon but potentially serious complication that can result in posterior capsular rupture and posterior dislocation of the crystalline lens. It is thought to occur because of a rapid increase in posterior fluid volume during hydrodissection, which can occur if fluid egress from the capsular space is impeded, usually from occlusion of the capsulorrhexis by the lens nucleus and cortex. Predisposing factors include posterior pole and mature cataract, long visual axis, and rapid and large volume hydrodissection. During laser fragmentation of the lens, intralenticular gas is produced with the potential to increase intracapsular volume.

Sudden wrinkling and movement of the lens capsule, tilting and instability of the lens following hydrodissection, or unexpected dislocation of the lens into the vitreous at the commencement of phacoemulsification suggests a posterior capsular rupture due to intraoperative CBS. Intraoperative pupillary block and subsequent rupture of the posterior capsule is thought to occur if the injected hydrodissection fluid does not flow freely around the lens within the capsular bag and out through the anterior capsulotomy and corneal incision. Rapid accumulation of fluid behind the lens-capsule complex can mimic a threatened expulsive hemorrhage. The eye becomes especially vulnerable when a highly cohesive ophthalmic viscosurgical device (OVD) is injected into the anterior chamber prior to hydrodissection. The presence of a normal capsule preoperatively strongly suggests intraoperative CBS; however, in cases of a weakened posterior capsule (eg, trauma, hypermature cataract, or congenital posterior polar cataract), spontaneous posterior capsular rupture can occur without intraoperative CBS.

PRECAUTIONS TO AVOID POSTERIOR CAPSULAR RUPTURE IN FEMTOSECOND LASER CATARACT SURGERY

Given the aforementioned potential risk factors, the authors recommend that the following intraoperative procedures be performed during laser-assisted cataract surgery:

- Reduce the OVD fill prior to anterior capsule removal to avoid overinflating the anterior chamber.

- Decompress the anterior chamber before and during hydrodissection by exerting pressure on the posterior lip of the corneal incision with the elbow of the cannula.

- Decompress the lens capsule during hydrodissection by elevating the anterior capsule with the tip of the hydrodissection cannula during injection.

- Inject the hydrodissection fluid slowly and titrate the volume based on the visibly expanding fluid wave.

- Use a prechopper or blunt-tipped, sideport instrument to split the hemispheres prior to hydrodissection to allow the gas and/or injected fluid to come forward.

- During gentle hydrodissection move the nucleus gently up, down, and around to let the gas bubble come forward to the anterior chamber. This is called the *rock & roll technique.*

CONCLUSION

Femtosecond laser treatment of the crystalline lens increases the safety, efficacy, and predictability of the surgery, though surgical skill and wisdom are still needed to avoid possible complications that might arise during lens surgery. During well-prepared surgeries (thorough patient information and selection, proper patient interface (PI) docking, well-designed and performed capsulotomy, lens fragmentation and liquefaction, corneal wound and astigmatic correction) the safety of refractive cataract surgery increases and the advantages of the premium lenses can be achieved and be of benefit to the patient. The danger of posterior capsular damage with meticulous hydrodissection is similar to traditional phacoemulsification. CBS can be avoided by the surgical technique mentioned previously; therefore, use of the femtosecond laser does not render the procedure more dangerous regarding posterior capsular damage. The integrated OCT imaging system proved to be an indispensable module in femtosecond laser cataract surgery. The OCT image guidance enhanced the safety of the procedure to avoid critical structures such as the posterior capsule.

REFERENCES

1. Osher RH, Cionni RJ. The torn posterior capsule: its intraoperative behavior, surgical management, and the long-term consequences. *J Cataract Refract Surg.* 1990;16:490-494.
2. Ota I, Miyake S, Miyake K. Dislocation of the lens nucleus into the vitreous cavity after standard hydrodissection. *Am J Ophthalmol.* 1996;121:706-708.
3. Osher RH, Yu BCY, Koch DD. Posterior polar cataracts: a predisposition to intraoperative posterior capsule rupture. *J Cataract Refract Surg.* 1990;16:157-162.
4. Chylack LT Jr, Wolfe JK, Singer DM, et al; for the Longitudinal Study of Cataract Study Group. The lens opacities classification system III. *Arch Ophthalmol.* 1993;111:831-836.
5. Marques FF, Marques DM, Osher RH, Osher JM. Fate of anterior capsule tears during cataract surgery. *J Cataract Refract Surg.* 2006;32:1638-1642.

6.   Unal M, Yücel I, Sarici A, et al. Phacoemulsification with topical anesthesia: resident experience. *J Cataract Refract Surg.* 2006;32:1361-1365.

7.   Nagy ZZ, Takacs A, Filkorn T, Sarayba M. Initial clinical evaluation of an intraocular femtosecond laser in cataract surgery. *J Refract Surg.* 2009;25:1053-1060.

8.   Nagy ZZ, Kranitz K, Takacs AI, Mihaltz K, Kovács I, Knorz MC. Comparison of intraocular lens decentration parameters after femtosecond and manual capsulotomies. *J Refract Surg.* 2011;27:564-569.

9.   Roberts TV, Sutton G, Lawless MA, Jindal-Bali S, Hodge C. Capsular block syndrome associated with femtosecond laser-assisted cataract surgery. *J Cataract Refract Surg.* 2011;37:2068-2070.

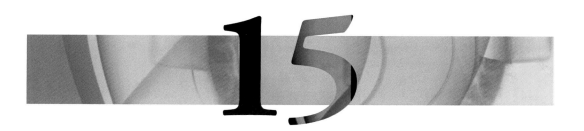

Management of
Dislocated Intraocular Lenses

Garry P. Condon, MD; Clement K. Chan, MD, FACS;
and Amar Agarwal, MS, FRCS, FRCOphth

Numerous advances in microsurgical techniques have led to safe and effective cataract surgery. Two of the current trends in the evolution of modern cataract techniques include increasingly smaller surgical incisions associated with phacoemulsification (eg, sub 1-mm incisions, such as in phakonit)[1], as well as the movement from retrobulbar and peribulbar anesthesia to topical anesthesia, and even techniques that do not require anesthesia.[2] Despite such advances, the malpositioning or dislocation of an intraocular lens (IOL) due to capsular rupture or zonular dehiscence remains an infrequent but important sight-threatening complication for contemporary cataract surgery. The key to preventing a poor visual outcome due to this complication is in proper management. Many highly effective surgical methods have been developed to manage a dislocated IOL. They include manipulating the IOL with perfluorocarbon liquids, scleral loop fixation using a snare, using 25-gauge IOL forceps, performing temporary haptic externalization, and managing the single-piece plate IOL and 2 simultaneous intraocular implants.[3-13]

MANAGEMENT OF A MALPOSITIONED INTRAOCULAR LENS

Disturbing visual symptoms such as diplopia, metamorphopsia, and hazy images are associated with a dislocated IOL. If not properly managed, a malpositioned IOL may also induce sight-threatening ocular complications including persistent cystoid macular edema (CME), intraocular hemorrhage, retinal breaks, and retinal detachment.

PERFLUOROCARBON LIQUIDS

Dr. David F. Chang popularized the use of perfluorocarbon liquids for the surgical treatment of various vitreoretinal disorders.[3] Due to their heavier-than-water properties and their ease of

Agarwal A.
*Posterior Capsular Rupture: A Practical Guide
to Prevention and Management* (pp 165-183).
© 2014 Taylor & Francis Group.

intraocular injection and removal,[14-17] perfluorocarbon liquids are highly effective for flattening detached retina, tamponading retinal tears, limiting intraocular hemorrhage, and floating dropped crystalline lens fragments and a dislocated IOL.[14-21] Due to their unique physical properties, perfluorocarbon liquids are well suited for floating dropped lens fragments and dislocated IOLs to insulate the underlying retina from damage. At the same time, the anterior displacement of the dislocated IOL by the perfluorocarbon liquids facilitates its removal or repositioning.[14-23]

ANTERIOR CHAMBER INTRAOCULAR LENSES

Dislocation of the anterior chamber IOL into the vitreous cavity is relatively infrequent compared to the posterior chamber IOL. However, the anterior chamber IOL may dislocate during trauma, particularly in the presence of a large-sector iridectomy. A subluxated or posteriorly dislocated anterior chamber IOL may simply be repositioned into the anterior chamber.[24,25] If the dislocated anterior chamber IOL is attached to formed vitreous or is sitting deep in the posterior vitreous cavity, an initial partial vitrectomy to eliminate the vitreoretinal traction is preferred before repositioning or removal of the anterior chamber IOL.[25] If there is any substantial anterior segment injury associated with the dislocation (eg, marked iridodialysis, large hyphema, or excessive angle damage), it is best to remove the dislocated anterior chamber IOL through a limbal incision.

OPENED-EYE OR EXTERNAL APPROACH

The opened-eye, or external, approach involves modifications of various suturing techniques for inserting an external primary or secondary posterior chamber IOL, sometimes in association with aphakic penetrating keratoplasty or with an IOL exchange in the absence of appropriate capsular or zonular support.[26-36] The suture material can be easily tied to the externally located IOL before its reinsertion. A relatively large limbal incision is required for the externalization and the subsequent reinsertion of the entire dislocated posterior chamber IOL.

CLOSED-EYE OR INTERNAL APPROACH: PARS PLANA TECHNIQUES

The closed-eye, or internal, approach avoids making a large surgical incision that may induce undesirable astigmatism or tissue injury. The integrity of the globe is maintained and the fluctuation of the IOP is minimized throughout the surgery. However, many internal techniques require the passage of sharp instruments or needles into the eye, which sometimes can be associated with the risk of injury to the intraocular structures. Relatively intricate intraocular maneuvers may also be involved. In recent years, a number of internal techniques for the repositioning the posterior chamber IOL with a pars plana approach have become increasingly popular.[4-11,21,22,37,38]

Scleral Loop Fixation

In 1991, Maguire et al[4] described the preparation of a 9-0 or 10-0 polypropylene suture loop by making a simple knot or a series of twists on the suture with a pair of microforceps. The same microforceps are used to grasp the suture adjacent to the suture loop for insertion through an anterior sclerotomy corresponding to the location of the ciliary sulcus after a partial pars plana vitrectomy to eliminate the vitreoretinal traction. The inserted suture loop is then used to engage

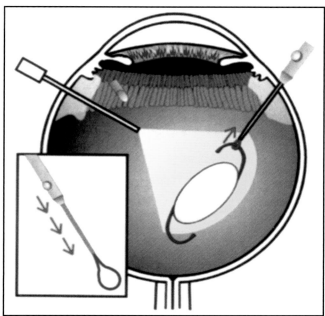

Figure 15-1. The Grieshaber snare consists of a 20-gauge tube and handle with a movable spring-loaded finger slide for adjusting the amount of a protruding polypropylene suture loop. The suture loop is inserted posteriorly to engage a dislocated haptic. The external portion of the suture loop is then cut free and guided through a 30-gauge needle for anchoring at the sclera, after the engaged haptic is pulled up against the anterior sclerotomy. (Reprinted with permission from CA Chan, Inc.)

one of the dislocated haptics for anchoring at the anterior sclerotomy. The same maneuver is repeated for the opposite haptic.

Grieshaber Snare

Grieshaber first manufactured a snare designed by Packo in the early 1990s. It consists of a 20-gauge tube and a handle with a movable, spring-loaded finger slide for adjusting the size of a protruding polypropylene loop. The distal portion of the tube with the polypropylene loop is inserted through an anterior sclerotomy for engaging a dislocated haptic in the vitreous cavity. After the looped haptic is pulled up against the anterior sclerotomy, the external portion of the polypropylene loop is cut free and guided through a 30-gauge needle for anchoring by the anterior sclerotomy (Figure 15-1). Little et al[5] reported the successful transscleral fixation of the dislocated posterior chamber IOL with the snare method in a series of cases in 1993.

MicroSurgical Technology (Redmond, WA) now has a 25-gauge suture snare, a design on which Condon has been working. It is curved and can be used easily via the sclera or cornea for up to 9-0 polypropylene suture.

25-Gauge Intraocular Lens Forceps

In 1994, Chang and Coll[6] introduced the 25-gauge IOL forceps. These passive-action forceps have smooth platforms at the distal end for grasping tissue or holding a suture and a small groove at the proximal end for gripping a haptic.[6] After a partial vitrectomy, a sharp 25-gauge, 5/8 inch needle is inserted through a scleral groove at 0.8 mm posterior to the corneoscleral limbus to create a tract for the 25-gauge forceps. The forceps holding a slip knot, or lasso, on a 10-0 polypropylene suture is then inserted through the grooved scleral incision into the eye for engaging an IOL haptic. After looping the haptic, the forceps are released from the suture and are used to regrasp the end of the haptic, thus preventing the suture from slipping off the haptic. After tightening the slip knot, the IOL is repositioned in the ciliary sulcus by anchoring the needle of the 10-0 polypropylene suture within the scleral groove (Figure 15-2). The same maneuver may be repeated for the opposite haptic, if necessary. The scleral groove is closed with an interrupted 10-0 nylon suture.

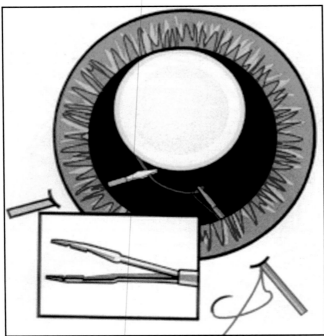

Figure 15-2. These 25-gauge Chang passive-action IOL forceps have smooth distal platforms for grasping tissues or sutures and a proximal groove for gripping a haptic. A slip knot is inserted through a paralimbal scleral groove incision to engage the haptic of the IOL. The forceps are then used to regrasp the distal end of the haptic to prevent slippage of the suture loop. After tightening the slip knot, the needle of the 10-0 polypropylene suture is anchored within the scleral groove for implant fixation in the ciliary sulcus. (Reprinted with permission from CA Chan, Inc.)

TEMPORARY HAPTIC EXTERNALIZATION

Chan first described the method of temporary haptic externalization in 1992.[7] Its main features involve temporary haptic externalization for suture placement after a pars plana vitrectomy followed by reinternalization of the haptics tied with 9-0 or 10-0 polypropylene sutures for secured anchoring by the anterior sclerotomies.[7] The details of this technique include the following[7,8]:

- A 3-port pars plana vitrectomy is performed for the removal of the anterior and central vitreous adjacent to the dislocated IOL to prevent any vitreoretinal traction during the process of manipulating the IOL.

- Two diametrically opposed limbal-based, partial thickness triangular scleral flaps are prepared along the horizontal meridians at 3 and 9 o'clock. Anterior sclerotomies within the beds under the scleral flaps are made at 1 to 1.5 mm from the limbus (Figure 15-3A). As an alternative to the scleral flaps, the anterior sclerotomies may be made within scleral grooves at 1 to 1.5 mm from the horizontal limbus.

- A fiberoptic light pipe is inserted through one of the posterior sclerotomies while a pair of fine, nonangled positive action forceps (eg, Grieshaber 612.8, Alcon Grieshaber Ltd, Schaffhausen, Switzerland) is inserted through the anterior sclerotomy of the opposing quadrant to engage one haptic of the dislocated IOL for temporary externalization (Figure 15-3B). A double-armed, 9-0 or 10-0 polypropylene suture is tied around the externalized haptic to make a secured knot. The same process is repeated for the other haptic after the surgeon switches the instruments to his or her opposite hand.

- The externalized haptics with the tied sutures are reinternalized through the corresponding anterior sclerotomies with the same forceps (Figure 15-3C). The surgeon anchors the internalized haptics securely in the ciliary sulcus by taking scleral bites with the external suture needles on the lips of the anterior sclerotomies. By adjusting the tension of the opposing

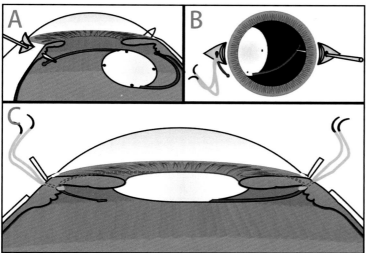

Figure 15-3. Temporary haptic externalization. (A) A pair of intraocular forceps without teeth is used to grasp one of the haptics for temporary externalization and placement of either 9-0 or 10-0 polypropylene suture. (B) The same is then performed for the opposite haptic. (C) The externalized haptics with the tied sutures are reinserted with the same forceps. (Reprinted with permission from CA Chan, Inc.)

sutures while tying the polypropylene suture knots by the anterior sclerotomies, the optic is centered behind the pupil, and the haptics are anchored in the ciliary sulcus.

Several important features of this technique include the following[7,8]:

- The horizontal meridians are chosen for the location of the anterior sclerotomies for easier manipulation of the forceps, haptics, and sutures during the repositioning process.

- The locations of the anterior sclerotomies determine the final position of the IOL. Previous anatomic studies have reported the ciliary sulcus to be between 0.46 and 0.8 mm from the limbus.[49] Thus, the distance of 1 to 1.5 mm from the limbus places the anterior sclerotomies close to the external surface of the ciliary sulcus. Making the anterior sclerotomies at less than 1 mm from the limbus increases the risk of injuring the anterior chamber angle or the iris root.

- The following steps are taken to ease the passage of the haptics through the anterior sclerotomies and reduce the chance of haptic breakage: (1) The anterior sclerotomies should have adequate size. If necessary, they may be widened before haptic reinternalization. (2) Fine, nonangled, positive action intraocular forceps are used for the haptic manipulation to give the surgeon maximal feel and control. Excessive pinching of the haptics is avoided during the passage of the haptics.

The following measures may also be taken to prevent the decentering and tilting of the IOL:

- The anterior sclerotomies are made at 180 degrees from each other.

- The sutures are tied at equal distance from the ends of both haptics.

- A 4-point fixation option can be performed. To enhance stability, 2 separate polypropylene sutures can be tied on each haptic, and the associated needles are anchored on the 2 "corners" of each anterior sclerotomy. This allows a stable configuration of 4-point fixation of the IOL.

This repositioning technique combines the best features of the external and internal approaches while avoiding any intricate and cumbersome intraocular manipulations. With the easy placement of the anchoring sutures[39-48] in an "opened" environment and the maintenance of the integrity of the globe in a "closed" environment, this technique allows a precise and secured fixation of the dislocated IOL in the ciliary sulcus on a consistent basis.[7-9]

Figure 15-4. The slippery plate implant may be lifted on its edge or hooked through a positioning hole with a lighted pick and then grasped with intraocular forceps for its repositioning or removal. (Reprinted with permission from CA Chan, Inc.)

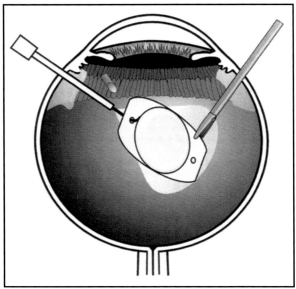

SINGLE-PIECE SILICONE PLATE INTRAOCULAR LENS

A lack of fibrous adhesion is noted between the lens capsule and the single-piece silicone IOL with plate haptics even years after its insertion into the capsular bag.[49-51] The "slippery" surface of the single-piece silicone plate implant makes it relatively mobile, even years after it has been placed. The silicone plate implant is fixated in the capsular bag by capsular contraction.[49-51] After implantation, there is fibrotic fusion of the anterior and posterior capsules, as well as capsular purse-stringing, due to anterior capsular contraction.[49-51] These effects induce the posterior bowing of the silicone plate implant against the posterior capsule, resulting in posterior capsular tightening and stretching.[49-51] Thus, any dehiscence of the capsular bag outside of the capsulorrhexis allows the release of the "built-up" tension and the expulsion of the implant through the dehiscence.[10,11,49-51] Frequently, further capsular contraction after a posterior neodymium-doped yttrium aluminum garnet (Nd:YAG) capsulotomy may then vault the single-piece silicone plate implant through the opening into the vitreous cavity in a delayed fashion.[10,11,49-51]

Previous reports have advocated repositioning the dislocated silicone plate implant anterior to the capsular remnants or in the ciliary sulcus.[10,11] Schneiderman et al[10] and Johnson and Schneiderman[11] described the technique of picking the slippery silicone plate implant off the retinal surface with a lighted pick. The surgeon extends the tip of the pick under the edge of the silicone plate implant to gently elevate it off the retinal surface. The elevated edge is then grasped with the intraocular forceps for the repositioning or removal of the implant. Alternatively, the plate implant may be brought anteriorly by hooking the lighted pick through one of its positioning holes and grasping with forceps at the anterior or mid-vitreous cavity (Figure 15-4).

Another method is to aspirate the plate implant with a soft-tip cannula. As discussed previously, perfluorocarbon liquids may also be used to float the dislocated plate implant. The single-piece silicone plate implant is designed for insertion into the capsular bag. Thus, repositioning the silicone plate implant anterior to the capsular remnants or in the ciliary sulcus tends to be unstable, particularly without the support of sutures.

No suturing methods (including the temporary haptic externalization technique described) work well for the single-piece silicone IOL with plate haptics. Temporary externalization of the bulky plate haptics of the silicone plate implant is awkward, and suture placement through its

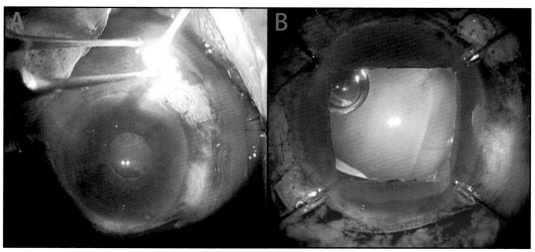

Figure 15-5. Chandelier illumination. (A) Chandelier illumination being fixed onto the trocar and cannula. (B) Note the bright vitreous cavity due to the chandelier illumination.

floppy surface tends to result in "cheese-wiring" of the implant. Frequently, the best approach for managing the dislocated single-piece silicone plate implant is its removal.

CHANDELIER ILLUMINATION

Visualization of the fundus during vitrectomy is done using chandelier illumination, which is the process by which a xenon light is fixed to a trocar cannula (Figure 15-5). This gives excellent illumination and one can perform a proper bimanual vitrectomy, as an endoilluminator is not necessary for the surgeon to hold in the hand. An inverter has to be used if one is using a wide-field lens. The Super Macula lens (Volk Optical, Mentor, OH) helps to give better stereopsis so that one will not have any difficulty holding the IOL with a diamond-tipped forceps. The surgeon can also use a noncontact viewing system, such as a binocular indirect ophthalmic microscope (BIOM). When the surgeon is using the chandelier illumination system, one hand can hold the IOL with the forceps and the other hand can hold a vitrectomy probe to cut the adhesions of the vitreous, thus doing a bimanual vitrectomy (Figure 15-6). One can also use 2 forceps to hold the lens, thus performing a handshake technique (Figure 15-7).

GLUED INTRAOCULAR LENS

The dislocated IOL can also be fixed using the glued IOL technique.[52-56] One advantage of this technique is the avoidance of suture-related complications of a sutured scleral-fixation IOL. Because the IOL haptic is tucked in the scleral tunnel, it prevents further movement of the haptic, thus reducing pseudophakodonesis and minimizing slippage and late redislocation. Although complete scleral wound healing with collagen fibrils may take up to 3 months because the haptic is snugly placed inside an intralamellar scleral tunnel, the IOL remains stable from the early postoperative period. This new method is further discussed in Chapter 12.

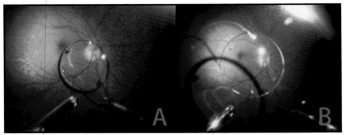

Figure 15-6. An intraoperative picture showing bimanual vitrectomy being performed in a completely dislocated IOL in the vitreous. Internal illumination, or chandelier illumination, is from the halogen light source attached with the infusion cannula. (A) An intraoperative picture showing bimanual vitrectomy being performed in a completely dislocated IOL in the vitreous. Note that one hand has a forceps to lift the IOL and the other hand has the vitrectomy probe to cut the adhesions of the vitreous. (B) Internal illumination is from the halogen light source attached to the infusion cannula.

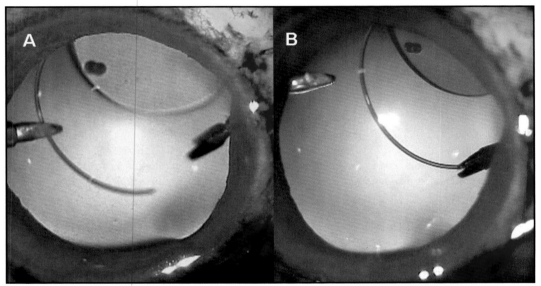

Figure 15-7. Handshake technique. Intravitreal forceps is used to hold the haptic while the IOL is brought to the pupillary plane.

Single-Piece, Nonfoldable Polymethyl Methacrylate Subluxated Intraocular Lens

It is a bit tricky to reposition a single-piece, nonfoldable polymethyl methacrylate (PMMA) IOL using the glued IOL technique because the haptics can break (Figure 15-8). Scleral flaps are created and vitrectomy is performed after fixing the infusion cannula. Using 2 glued IOL forceps and the handshake technique, each haptic is then externalized through opposite sclerotomies under the scleral flaps. They are then tucked and glued in the Scharioth tunnels.

Subluxated Capsular Bag–Intraocular Lens Complex

The subluxated capsular bag-IOL complex is tricky to handle (Figure 15-9). In such cases, there may be thick Soemmering's rings. Vitrectomy of these can be done, but sometimes they are quite

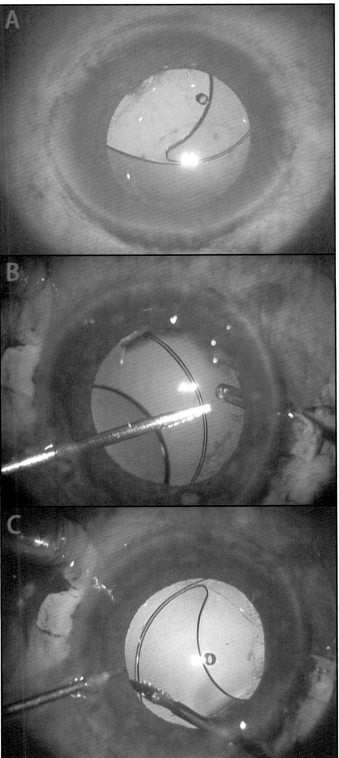

Figure 15-8. Management of a subluxated single-piece PMMA nonfoldable IOL. (A) Subluxated single-piece PMMA IOL. (B) Vitrectomy performed. Note one haptic is held with the glued IOL forceps to prevent the IOL from falling down while vitrectomy is done. (C) One haptic is caught with the glued IOL forceps.

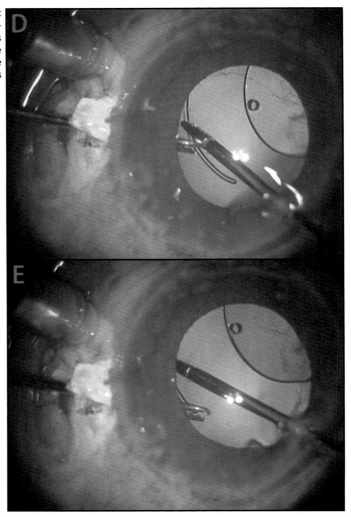

Figure 15-8 (continued). Management of a subluxated single-piece PMMA non-foldable IOL. (D) The second forceps is passed through the sclerotomy under the scleral flap to grab the haptic using the handshake technique. (E) The haptic tip is grasped to externalize the haptic.

thick and can fall into the vitreous cavity. In the case of dangling IOLs, the complex is explanted through a scleral tunnel incision. Vitrectomy is then performed and a 3-piece IOL is glued into place.

Glued Endocapsular Ring

If the IOL is not dangling, the dislocated bag-IOL complex can also be transsclerally fixated by using a glued endocapsular ring as described by Dr. Soosan Jacob (see Chapter 5). The haptic of the ring is exteriorized through a sclerotomy under a scleral flap and tucked into an intrascleral Scharioth tunnel created at the edge of the scleral flap. Fibrin glue is used to seal the flap and conjunctiva.

Single-Piece, Foldable Intraocular Lens

The single-piece, foldable IOL cannot be fixed and glued, as the haptic is not suitable. The haptics in a single-piece, foldable IOL are too flexible and too thick to tuck and glue. In such cases, depending on the extent of subluxation, the IOL is either explanted and a new 3-piece IOL fixed

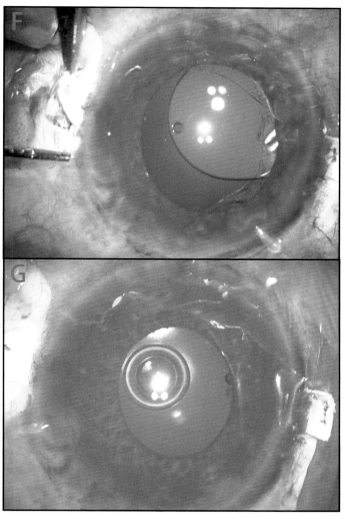

Figure 15-8 (continued). Management of a subluxated single-piece PMMA non-foldable IOL. (F) The haptic externalized. One should be careful when doing this maneuver in a single-piece, nonfoldable PMMA IOL, as the haptic can break. (G) Both haptics are externalized and tucked. Glue will then be applied. Note the well-centered IOL.

with the glued IOL technique or the bag-IOL complex stabilized with a glued endocapsular ring is implanted. This has the advantage of avoiding the use of sutures, thus giving greater stability and longevity.

IRIS SUTURING OF THE INTRAOCULAR LENS

The ideal location for the placement of an IOL in the absence of capsular support remains controversial. Methods for scleral fixation of posterior chamber IOLs are relatively complex, may result in lens tilt, and rely on the placement of permanent transscleral sutures that can have late complications including suture breakage with IOL dislocation and suture-related endophthalmitis. Since 1976, the McCannel[57] retrievable suture technique has proven successful for repositioning dislocated posterior chamber IOLs. Repositioning of a dislocated posterior chamber IOL using McCannel sutures for iris fixation can be reliable and safe, and at the same time is advantageous in avoiding a large incision and external sutures.[57-65]

Figure 15-9. Management of a sub-luxated capsular bag-IOL complex. (A) Subluxated capsular bag-IOL complex. Measure the WTW diameter of the cornea, and if the horizontal is more than 11 mm, perform a vertical glued IOL implantation. (B) Scleral flaps are made, the infusion is fixed, and vitrectomy done. One hand holds the haptic with a glued IOL forceps to prevent the bag-IOL complex from falling down. (C) Explantation of the bag-IOL complex through a sclera tunnel incision. One can perform a vitrectomy and chew up the bag, but in some cases there are thick Soemmering's rings, which are sometimes difficult to chew and can fall down onto the retina. In such cases, it might be more prudent to explant the entire complex.

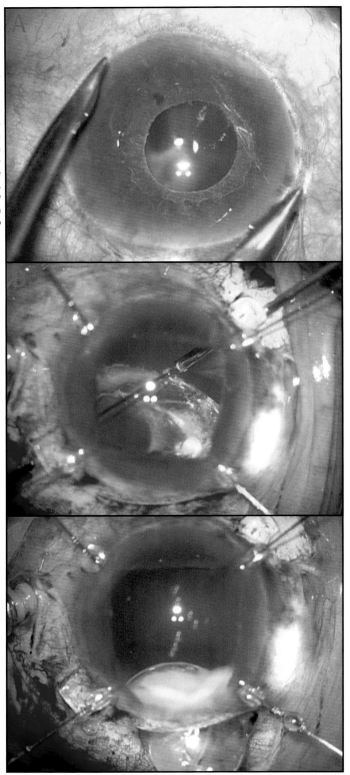

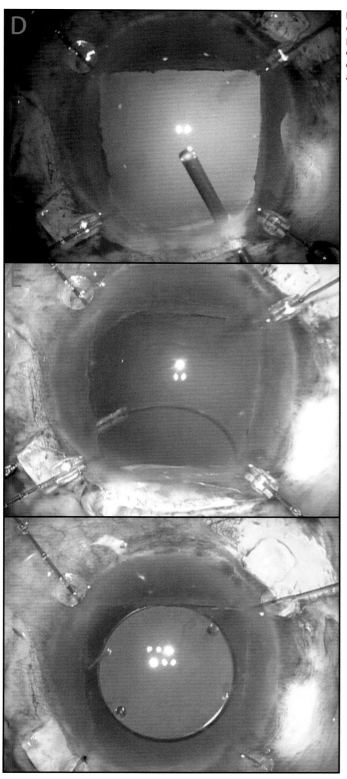

Figure 15-9 (continued). Management of a subluxated capsular bag-IOL complex. (D) Vitrectomy. (E) Glued IOL started with a 3-piece IOL. (F) Haptics are externalized and tucked. Finally glue is applied.

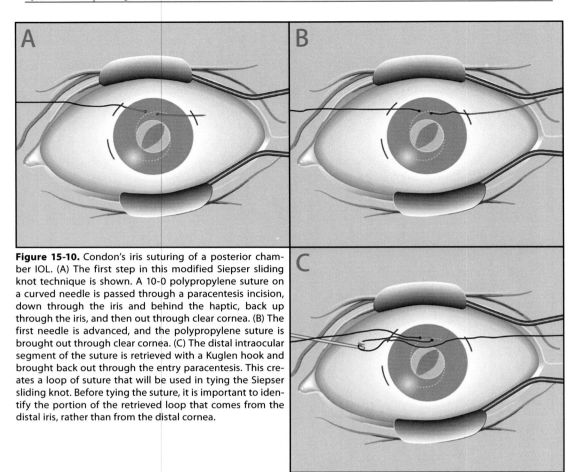

Figure 15-10. Condon's iris suturing of a posterior chamber IOL. (A) The first step in this modified Siepser sliding knot technique is shown. A 10-0 polypropylene suture on a curved needle is passed through a paracentesis incision, down through the iris and behind the haptic, back up through the iris, and then out through clear cornea. (B) The first needle is advanced, and the polypropylene suture is brought out through clear cornea. (C) The distal intraocular segment of the suture is retrieved with a Kuglen hook and brought back out through the entry paracentesis. This creates a loop of suture that will be used in tying the Siepser sliding knot. Before tying the suture, it is important to identify the portion of the retrieved loop that comes from the distal iris, rather than from the distal cornea.

The Condon Technique

A 1-mm peripheral paracentesis stab incision is made 180 degrees away from the incision site. In cases of primary posterior chamber IOL implantation, the lens optic is folded across the 10 to 4 o'clock meridians and is held in a Fine inserter II instrument (05-2339-R; Rhein Medical, Tampa, FL). The dislocated posterior chamber IOL is brought anteriorly. Viscoelastics are used to deepen the chamber. The haptics remain behind the iris while the optic is captured by the miotic pupil and stabilized. Additional viscoelastic is then injected to reform the chamber and to better delineate the haptic location.

Another paracentesis is then made to allow passage of a 10-0 polypropylene suture on a curved PC-7 needle (Alcon Laboratories, Fort Worth, TX) through the paracentesis, down through the iris and behind the haptic, back up through the iris, and then out through clear cornea (Figure 15-10A). Another curved needle is then passed in the same fashion under the opposite haptic. The first needle is then advanced and the suture is brought out through clear cornea (Figure 15-10B). The distal intraocular segment of the suture is retrieved with a Kuglen hook and brought back out through the entry paracentesis, creating a loop (Figure 15-10C). To secure the haptics, a modified Siepser sliding knot is created. Before tying the suture, it is important to identify the portion of

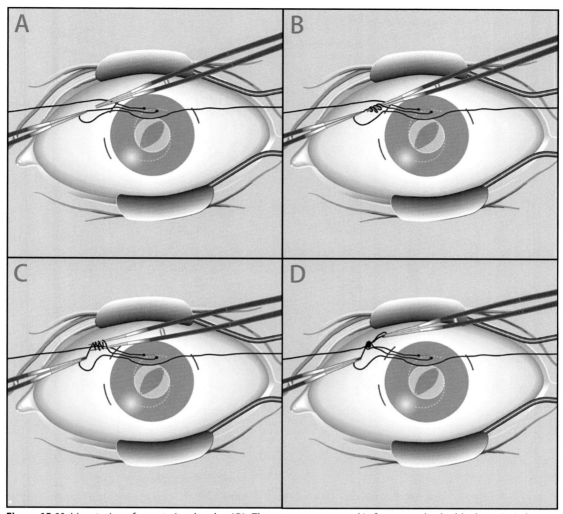

Figure 15-11. Iris suturing of a posterior chamber IOL. The sutures are grasped in forceps and a double throw is tied.

the retrieved loop that comes from the distal iris, rather than from the distal cornea. The proximal portion of the retrieved loop of suture is tied to the trailing suture segment with a double throw (Figure 15-11).

The trailing suture segment is then stabilized, traction is placed on the distal suture segment, and the knot is gathered and pulled into the anterior chamber to secure the haptic (Figure 15-12). The distal segment is retrieved again and used to create the next throw, which can be a single throw in the opposite direction to the first. In this step, it is important to identify the side of the retrieved loop coming from the knot. Before tying the first double-throw suture knot, the surgeon must verify that he or she has the portion of the retrieved loop coming from the distal iris, rather than the distal cornea.

The same technique is used for suture fixation of the other haptic. After both sutures are tightened, the ends are trimmed with intraocular scissors and the optic is prolapsed into the posterior chamber using a spatula. Any slight ovalization of the pupil that is observed at the end of the procedure can be reduced with gentle traction by the spatula at the suture sites.

Figure 15-12. Iris suturing of a posterior chamber IOL. (A) The trailing suture segment is stabilized. (B) Traction is placed on the distal suture segment. (C) The knot is gathered and pulled into the anterior chamber to secure the haptic.

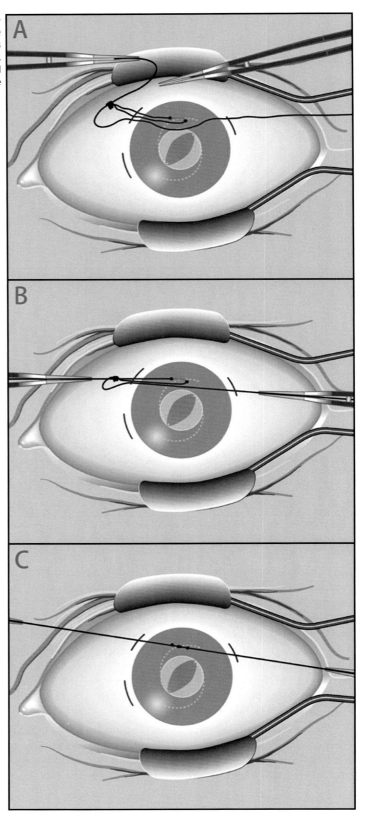

CONCLUSION

The management of a malpositioned or dislocated intraocular implant is best accomplished via modern pars plana technology. The basic principles of management include initial anterior and posterior vitrectomy to eliminate any vitreous traction followed by the use of various intraocular microforceps, and various techniques to engage the dislocated IOL for its removal or repositioning.

REFERENCES

1. Agarwal A, Agarwal A, Agarwal S, Narang P, Narang S. Phakonit: phacoemulsification through a 0.9 mm corneal incision. *J Cataract Refract Surg.* 2001;27(10):1548-1552.
2. Pandey SK, Werner L, Apple DJ, Agarwal A, Agarwal A, Agarwal S. No-anesthesia clear corneal phacoemulsification versus topical and topical plus intracameral anesthesia. Randomized clinical trial. *J Cataract Refract Surg.* 2001;27(10):1643-1650.
3. Chang S. Perfluorocarbon liquids in vitreo-retinal surgery. *International Ophthalmology Clinics.* 1992;32(2):153-163.
4. Maguire AM, Blumenkranz MS, Ward TG, Winkelman JZ. Scleral loop fixation for posteriorly dislocated intraocular lenses: operative technique and long-term results. *Arch Ophthalmol.* 1991;109:1754-1758.
5. Little BC, Rosen PH, Orr G, Aylward GW. Trans-scleral fixation of dislocated posterior chamber intraocular lenses using a 9-0 microsurgical polypropylene snare. *Eye.* 1993;7:740-743.
6. Chang S, Coll GE. Surgical techniques for repositioning a dislocated intraocular lens, repair of iridodialysis, and secondary intraocular lens implantation using innovative 25-gauge forceps. *Am J Ophthalmol.* 1995;119:165-174.
7. Chan CK. An improved technique for management of dislocated posterior chamber implants. *Ophthalmology.* 1992;99:51-57.
8. Chan CK, Agarwal A, Agarwal S, Agarwal A. Management of dislocated intraocular implants. *Ophthalmology Clinics of North America.* 2001;14(4):681-693.
9. Thach AB, Dugel PU, Sipperley JO, et al. Outcome of sulcus fixation of dislocated PCIOL's using temporary externalization of the haptics. Paper presented at the American Academy of Ophthalmology Annual Meeting; November 10, 1998; New Orleans, LA.
10. Schneiderman TE, Johnson MW, Smiddy WE, et al. Surgical management of posteriorly dislocated silicone plate haptic intraocular lenses. *Am J Ophthalmol.* 1997;123:629-635.
11. Johnson MW, Schneiderman TE. Surgical management of posteriorly dislocated silicone plate intraocular lenses. *Curr Opin Ophthalmol.* 1998;9:11-15.
12. Williams DF, Del Piero EJ, Ferrone PJ, et al. Management of complications in eyes containing two intraocular lenses. *Ophthalmology.* 1998;105:2017-2022.
13. Wong KL, Grabow HB. Simplified technique to remove posteriorly dislocated lens implants. *Arch Ophthalmol.* 2001;119:273-274.
14. Glaser BM, Carter JB, Kuppermann BD, Michels RG. Perfluoro-octane in the treatment of giant retinal tears with proliferative vitreo-retinopathy. *International Ophthalmology Clinics.* 1992;32(2):1-14.
15. Nabih M, Peyman GA, Clark LC Jr, et al. Experimental evaluation of perfluorophenanthrene as a high specific gravity vitreous substitute: a preliminary report. *Ophthalmic Surg.* 1989;20:286-293.
16. Blinder KJ, Peyman GA, Paris CL, et al. Vitreon, a new perfluorocarbon. *Br J Opthalmol.* 1991;75:240-244.
17. Shapiro MJ, Resnick KI, Kim SH, Weinberg A. Management of the dislocated crystalline lens with a perfluorocarbon liquid. *Am J Ophthalmol.* 1991;112:401-405.
18. Liu K, Peyman GA, Chen M, Chang K. Use of high density vitreous substitute in the removal of posteriorly dislocated lenses or intraocular lenses. *Ophthalmic Surg.* 1991;22:503-507.
19. Lewis H, Blumenkranz MS, Chang S. Treatment of dislocated crystalline lens and retinal detachment with perfluorocarbon liquids. *Retina.* 1992;12:299-304.
20. Rowson NJ, Bacon AS, Rosen PH. Perfluorocarbon heavy liquids in the management of posterior dislocation of the lens nucleus during phacoemulsification. *Br J Ophthalmol.* 1992;176(3):169-170.
21. Greve MD, Peyman GA, Mehta NJ, Millsap CM. Use of perfluoroperhydrophenanthrene in the management of posteriorly dislocated crystalline and intraocular lenses. *Ophthalmic Surg.* 1993;24(9):593-597.
22. Lewis H, Sanchez G. The use of perfluorocarbon liquids in the repositioning of posteriorly dislocated intraocular lenses. *Ophthalmology.* 1993;100:1055-1059.
23. Elizalde J. Combined use of perfluorocarbon liquids and viscoelastics for safer surgical approach to posterior lens luxation. Poster Presented at the Vitreous Society 17th Annual Meeting; September 21-25, 1999; Rome, Italy.

24. Flynn HW Jr. Pars plana vitrectomy in the management of subluxated and posteriorly dislocated intraocular lenses. *Graefes Arch Clin Exp Ophthalmol.* 1987;225:169-172.

25. Flynn HW Jr, Buus D, Culbertson WW. Management of subluxated and posteriorly dislocated intraocular lenses using pars plana vitrectomy instrumentation. *J Cataract Refract Surg.* 1990;16:51-56.

26. Stark WJ, Goodman G, Goodman D, Gottsch J. Posterior chamber intraocular lens implantation in the absence of posterior capsular support. *Ophthalmic Surg.* 1988;19:240-243.

27. Hu BV, Shin DH, Gibbs KA, Hong YJ. Implantation of posterior chamber lens in the absence of posterior capsular and zonular support. *Arch Ophthalmol.* 1988;106:416-420.

28. Shin DH, Hu BV, Hong YJ, Gibbs KA. Posterior chamber lens implantation in the absence of posterior capsular support. *Ophthalmic Surg.* 1988;19:606-607.

29. Dahan E. Implantation in the posterior chamber without capsular support. *J Cataract Refract Surg.* 1989;15:339-342.

30. Pannu JS. A new suturing technique for ciliary sulcus fixation in the absence of posterior capsule. *Ophthalmic Surg.* 1988;19:751-754.

31. Spigelman AV, Lindstrom RL, Nichols BD, et al. Implantation of a posterior chamber lens without capsular support during penetrating keratoplasty or as a secondary lens implant. *Ophthalmic Surg.* 1988;19:396-398.

32. Drews RC. Posterior chamber lens implantation during keratoplasty without posterior lens capsule support. *Cornea.* 1987;6:38-40.

33. Wong SK, Stark WJ, Gottsch SD, et al. Use of posterior chamber lenses in pseudophakic bullous keratopathy. *Arch Ophthalmol.* 1987;105:856-858.

34. Waring GO III, Stulting RD, Street D. Penetrating keratoplasty for pseudophakic corneal edema with exchange of intraocular lenses. *Arch Ophthalmol.* 1987;105:58-62.

35. Shin DH. Implantation of a posterior chamber lens without capsular support during penetrating keratoplasty or as a secondary lens. *Ophthalmic Surg.* 1988;19:755-756.

36. Lindstrom RL, Harris WS, Lyle WA. Secondary and exchange posterior chamber lens implantation. *J Am Intraocul Implant Soc.* 1982;8:353-356.

37. Bloom SM, Wyszynski RE, Brucker AJ. Scleral fixation suture for dislocated posterior chamber intraocular lens. *Ophthalmic Surg.* 1990;21:851-854.

38. Friedberg MA, Pilkerton AR. A new technique for repositioning and fixating a dislocated intraocular lens. *Arch Ophthalmol.* 1992;110:413-415.

39. Jacobi KW, Krey H. Surgical management of intraocular lens dislocation into the vitreous: case report. *J Am Intraocul Implant Soc.* 1983;9:58-59.

40. Mittra RA, Connor TB, Han DP, et al. Removal of dislocated intraocular lenses using pars plana vitrectomy with placement of an open-loop, flexible anterior chamber lens. *Ophthalmology.* 1998;105:1011-1014.

41. McCannel MA. A retrievable suture idea for anterior uveal problems. *Ophthalmic Surg.* 1976;7(2):98-103.

42. Stark WJ, Bruner WE. Management of posteriorly dislocated intraocular lenses. *Ophthalmic Surg.* 1980;11:495-497.

43. Sternberg P Jr, Michels RG. Treatment of dislocated posterior chamber intraocular lenses. *Arch Ophthalmol.* 1986;104:1391-1393.

44. Girard LJ. Pars plana phacoprosthesis (aphakic intraocular implant): a preliminary report. *Ophthalmic Surg.* 1981;12:19-22.

45. Girard LJ, Nino N, Wesson M, et al. Scleral fixation of a subluxated posterior chamber intraocular lens. *J Cataract Refract Surg.* 1988;14:326-327.

46. Smiddy WE. Dislocated posterior chamber intraocular lens. A new technique of management. *Arch Ophthalmol.* 1989;107:1678-1680.

47. Campo RV, Chung KD, Oyakawa RT. Pars plana vitrectomy in the management of dislocated posterior chamber lenses. *Am J Ophthalmol.* 1989;108:529-534.

48. Anand R, Bowman RW. Simplified technique for suturing dislocated posterior chamber intraocular lens to the ciliary sulcus. *Arch Ophthalmol.* 1990;108:1205-1206.

49. Milauskas AT. Posterior capsule opacification after silicone lens implantation and its management. *J Cataract Refract Surg.* 1987;3:644-648.

50. Milauskas AT. Capsular bag fixation of one-piece silicone lenses. *J Cataract Refract Surg.* 1990;16:583-586.

51. Joo CK, Shin JA, Kim JH. Capsular opening contraction after continuous curvilinear capsulorrhexis and intraocular lens implantation. *J Cataract Refract Surg.* 1996;22:585-590.

52. Agarwal A, Kumar DA, Jacob S, Baid C, Agarwal A, Srinivasan S. Fibrin glue-assisted sutureless posterior chamber intraocular lens implantation in eyes with deficient posterior capsules. *J Cataract Refract Surg.* 2008;34:1433-1438.

53. Prakash G, Ashokumar D, Jacob S, Kumar KS, Agarwal A, Agarwal A. Anterior segment optical coherence tomography-aided diagnosis and primary posterior chamber intraocular lens implantation with fibrin glue in traumatic phacocele with scleral perforation. *J Cataract Refract Surg.* 2009;35:782-784.

54. Prakash G, Jacob S, Kumar DA, et al. Femtosecond-assisted keratoplasty with fibrin glue-assisted sutureless posterior chamber lens implantation: new triple procedure. *J Cataract Refract Surg.* 2009;35:973-979.

55. Agarwal A, Kumar DA, Jacob S, Prakash G, Agarwal A. Reply to letter: Fibrin glue–assisted sutureless posterior chamber intraocular lens implantation in eyes with deficient posterior capsules. *J Cataract Refract Surg.* 2009;35:795-796.

56. Nair V, Kumar DA, Prakash G, Jacob S, Agarwal A, Agarwal A. Bilateral spontaneous in-the-bag anterior subluxation of PC IOL managed with glued IOL technique: a case report. *Eye Contact Lens.* 2009;35:215-217.

57. McCannel MA. A retrievable suture idea for anterior uveal problems. *Ophthalmic Surg.* 1976;7:98-103.

58. Schein OD, Kenyon KR, Steinert RF, et al. A randomized trial of intraocular lens fixation techniques with penetrating keratoplasty. *Ophthalmology.* 1993;100:1437-1443.

59. Wagoner MD, Cox TA, Ariyasu RG, et al. Intraocular lens implantation in the absence of capsular support: a report by the American Academy of Ophthalmology. *Ophthalmology.* 2003;110:840-859.

60. Siepser SB. The closed chamber slipping suture technique for iris repair. *Ann Ophthalmol.* 1994;26:71-72.

61. Condon GP. Simplified small-incision peripheral iris fixation of an AcrySof intraocular lens in the absence of capsule support. *J Cataract Refract Surg.* 2003;29:1663-1667.

62. Condon GP, Ahmed I. No capsule, no problem: iris suture fixation of foldable acrylic IOLs. Video presented at the ASCRS/ASOA Symposium on Cataract, IOL and Refractive Surgery; May 1, 2004; San Diego, CA.

63. Condon GP, Ahmed IK, Masket S, et al. Iris fixation of foldable PC IOLs with modified McCannel slip-knot suture. Presented at the ASCRS/ASOA Symposium on Cataract, IOL and Refractive Surgery; April 14, 2003; San Francisco, CA.

64. Stutzman RD, Stark WJ. Surgical technique for suture fixation of an acrylic intraocular lens in the absence of capsule support. *J Cataract Refract Surg.* 2003;29:1658-1662.

65. Chang DF. Siepser slipknot for McCannel iris-suture fixation of subluxated intraocular lenses. *J Cataract Refract Surg.* 2004;30:1170–1176.

This chapter has been adapted with permission from Chan CK, Schultz GR. Management of dislocated implants by the vitreoretinal approach. In: Agarwal S, Agarwal A, Sachdev MS, et al (eds). *Phacoemulsification, Laser Cataract Surgery and Foldable IOLs.* 2nd ed. Jaypee Brothers Medical Publishers (P) Ltd; New Delhi; 2000:424-428.

16

Corneal Damage and Posterior Capsular Rupture

Soosan Jacob, MS, FRCS, DNB, MNAMS and
Amar Agarwal, MS, FRCS, FRCOphth

Posterior capsular rupture can result in various complications including corneal damage.[1-32] Corneal damage could be due to ensuing vitreous loss, manipulations by the surgeon, or the implantation of a suboptimal intraocular lens (IOL) in terms of its design, material, or location. It is important for the surgeon to understand the ramifications of corneal damage that can occur and how to manage it.

DESCEMET'S MEMBRANE DETACHMENT

Descemet's membrane detachment is a complication occasionally faced after surgery.[7,8] Various techniques have been proposed as treatment for Descemet's membrane detachment including observation,[9] viscoelastic injection,[10] air injection, the use of long-acting intracameral gas,[11,12] and insertion of transcorneal mattress sutures.[13] A detached Descemet's membrane can be diagnosed on slit-lamp examination as a clear optical space between the stroma and the Descemet's membrane.

Trypan blue dye may be injected into the anterior chamber to stain the Descemet's membrane and aid in visualization. The anterior chamber is then irrigated with balanced salt solution (BSS) to wash away excess trypan blue and to study the dynamics of the detached Descemet's membrane (Figure 16-1). An air bubble is then injected to appose the Descemet's membrane to the corneal stroma. Gases, such as sulphur hexafluoride (SF6) or perfluoropropane (C3F8), can also be used in more severe or long-standing cases.

Agarwal A.
Posterior Capsular Rupture: A Practical Guide
to Prevention and Management (pp 185-197).
© 2014 Taylor & Francis Group.

Figure 16-1. A stripped Descemet's membrane is shown. It is typically seen near incisions and it lies loose, floating in the anterior chamber. It may have a crumpled or rolled-up edge with an undulating appearance on anterior segment optical coherence tomography (OCT), and it flutters on irrigating the anterior chamber with BSS.

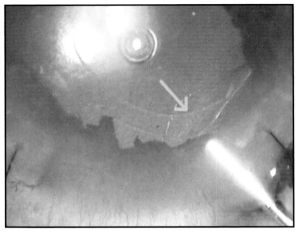

NEW CLASSIFICATION OF DESCEMET'S MEMBRANE DETACHMENT

Based on pathological features, Descemet's membrane detachment had been classified in 1928 by Samuels as active (pushed back) or passive (pulled back and torn away) due to differences in elasticity between the parenchyma and the glass membrane.[6] Samuels also stated that this classification was more relevant pathologically and no great importance could be ascribed to these forms of detachment from the surgical standpoint. Descemet's membrane detachment has also been previously classified as planar (less than 1-mm gap between Descemet's membrane and stroma) or nonplanar (more than 1-mm gap between Descemet's membrane and stroma) based on morphology.[7]

Dr. Soosan Jacob proposed a new classification of Descemet's membrane detachment based on the clinicomorphological, etiological, tomographic, and intraoperative features and she proposed a new treatment algorithm for Descemet's membrane detachment based on its classification. This classification of Descemet's membrane detachment is analogous to the classification of retinal detachment. The Descemet's membrane is a vital layer of the cornea and is necessary for maintaining the clarity of the cornea, just as the neurosensory retina is required for visual perception. As a retinal detachment can be rhegmatogenous retinal detachment (RRD [secondary to hole, tear, or dialysis]), tractional retinal detachment (TRD), or bullous/exudative retinal detachment, the authors would like to classify Descemet's membrane detachment into rhegmatogenous Descemet's detachment (RDD), tractional Descemet's detachment (TDD), bullous Descemet's detachment (BDD), or complex Descemet's detachment (CDD) (Table 16-1).

An RDD generally occurs as an intraoperative event when there is a break in the Descemet's membrane, with fluid accumulation between the Descemet's membrane and overlying stroma. Analogous to an RRD, an RDD can be secondary to a hole (eg, a double anterior chamber following perforation during deep anterior lamellar keratoplasty) or a tear (eg, Descemet's membrane detachment occurring during insertion of blunt instruments or IOL implantation during phacoemulsification). RDD can also occur secondary to a dialysis of the Descemet's membrane from its attachment at the Schwalbe's line, a complication that is sometimes seen during trabeculotomy, punch insertion in trabeculectomy, anterior chamber maintainer insertion, or if stripping of the Descemet's membrane accidentally extends toward the periphery during Descemet's membrane endothelial keratoplasty (DMEK).

TABLE 16-1. DIFFERENTIATING FEATURES OF TYPES OF DESCEMET'S MEMBRANE DETACHMENTS

	RHEGMATOGENOUS DESCEMET'S DETACHMENT	TRACTIONAL DESCEMET'S DETACHMENT	BULLOUS DESCEMET'S DETACHMENT	COMPLEX DESCEMET'S DETACHMENT
Time of Onset	Mostly intraoperative	Mostly postoperative	Secondary to disease process; sometimes intraoperative	Intra- or postoperative
History	History of surgery	History of inflammation, trauma, or surgery	History specific to underlying etiology	Generally there is a history of surgery
Cause	Tear, hole, or dialysis	Incarceration of Descemet's membrane in inflammation/fibrosis/ peripheral anterior synechiae/within the graft host junction/in wound/suture with subsequent contraction. Long standing RDD becoming adherent to intraocular contents with secondary TDD	Disease process, infection, or inflammation. Intraoperative complication (eg, blood or accidental injection of viscoelastic)	Poorly positioned DMEK graft. Combination of other DDs
Clinical Findings	Undulating membrane lying loose in the anterior chamber. Folds present. Undulating movements seen on irrigating anterior chamber with BSS	Undulating membrane lying between points of attachment. folds. Immobile or sharp, fluttering movements seen on forcible irrigation with BSS. Stretched out tight like a trampoline between two points of attachment. No break	Convex membrane bulging into the anterior chamber with no break	Complex configurations or combination features of others
Anterior Segment OCT	Undulating linear hyper-reflective signal in the anterior chamber. Arc length of overlying stroma is similar to length of detached Descemet's membrane	Straight taut linear hyper-reflective signal between two points of attachment. Arc length of cornea is more than length of detached Descemet's membrane	Convex hyper-reflective signal bulging into AC from overlying stroma. Space filled with exudate, pus, blood, viscoelastic, air, etc	Complex configurations or combination features of others
Prognosis	Good if residual endothelial function adequate	Good if residual endothelial function adequate	Prognosis depending on cause	Depending on cause

Figure 16-2. A taut Descemet's membrane detachment is seen stretched out between points of attachment on anterior segment OCT. It appears as a taut, linear hyper-reflection. Intraoperatively, it does not show much movement on irrigating the anterior chamber with BSS.

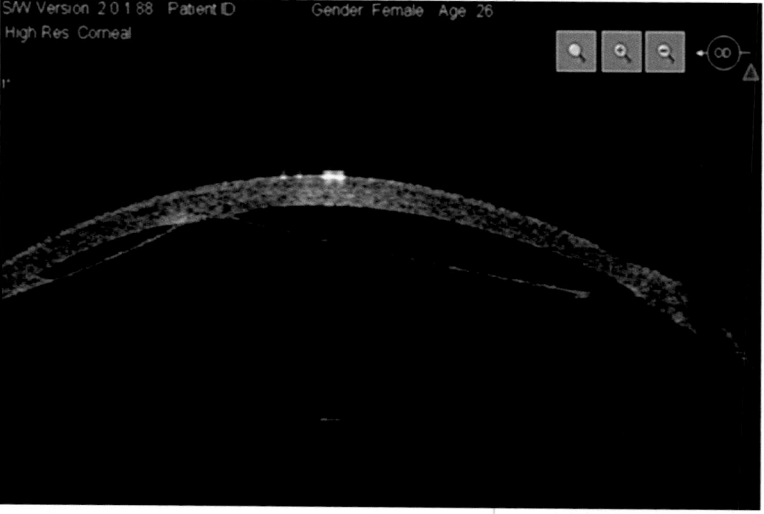

The Descemet's membrane may also become detached secondary to an inflammatory/fibrotic process, resulting in TDD, which is analogous to a TRD. This could be secondary to incarceration of the Descemet's membrane in an inflammatory process (eg, in peripheral anterior synechiae or within the graft host junction in large diameter grafts) or secondary to incarceration in a wound or suture with subsequent contraction, resulting in a TDD. A long-standing RDD could also sometimes adhere to intraocular contents with secondary fibrosis, thus turning into a TDD. A BDD can occur secondary to a disease process, such as posterior corneal abscess, tumor, infection, or inflammation (analogous to bullous retinal detachment). In this type of Descemet's membrane detachment, a separation and convex bulging of the Descemet's membrane into the anterior chamber occurs in the absence of a break in the Descemet's membrane. The space in between the stroma and the Descemet's membrane is filled with pus, exudates, fluid, viscoelastic, or air, depending on the cause of BDD. This configuration of Descemet's membrane can also be seen as part of the Anwar's big bubble technique in deep anterior lamellar keratoplasty, which detaches the Descemet's membrane from the stroma and sometimes occurs from accidental injection of viscoelastic into the pre-Descemetic space.[33] Clinically, an RDD is usually seen as an undulating membrane lying loose in the anterior chamber. It may also be scrolled or crumpled, depending on the extent of detachment. It has folds and is mobile, similar to an RRD. On the other hand, a TDD is stretched out tight, like a trampoline, between the points of attachment. It has no folds and is not mobile. A BDD is seen as a convex membrane bulging into the anterior chamber, similar to a bullous retinal detachment. A complex Descemet's detachment shows complex folds or scrolls or shows combination features of others and can be seen sometimes in a poorly attached DMEK graft.

ANTERIOR SEGMENT OPTICAL COHERENCE TOMOGRAPHY FEATURES

In all cases of Descemet's membrane detachment, there is generally overlying corneal epithelial and stromal edema which may make visualization difficult. In this case, the anterior segment OCT is useful for diagnosing this condition as well as differentiating between various types of Descemet's membrane detachment. An RDD is seen as an undulating linear hyper-reflective signal in the anterior chamber, whereas a TDD is seen as a straight, taut, linear signal between 2 points of attachment (Figure 16-2). In TDD, the arc length of the cornea, if measured, is found to be more than the length of the detached Descemet's membrane, unlike in RDD, where the arc length of the overlying corneal stroma is similar to the length of the detached Descemet's membrane. A BDD is seen as a convex, hyper-reflective signal bulging into the anterior chamber from the overlying stroma, with the space in between filled with exudate, pus, fluid, or air, depending on the cause of Descemet's membrane detachment. A CDD shows complex configurations on anterior segment OCT.

Intraoperatively, TDD can be verified by its more immobile nature and the absence of the typical undulating movement that is associated with an RDD on irrigating the anterior chamber with BSS. A taut Descemet's membrane does not move with the undulations seen in an RDD, although it might show some sharp, small, fluttery movements on forcible irrigation with BSS.

RELAXING DESCEMETOTOMY

Relaxing retinotomy is an established surgical technique in vitreoretinal surgery for periretinal traction and retinal foreshortening that does not allow the retina to settle down. Similar traction on the Descemet's membrane secondary to inflammation or fibrosis or the Descemet's membrane becoming incarcerated in a wound or suture leading to a TDD may not respond to the classic management strategies for Descemet's membrane detachment. Injecting air or long-acting gas into the anterior chamber in an eye with TDD will not appose it to the corneal stroma because of the foreshortening. Dr. Jacob developed a technique called *relaxing descemetotomy*, which is based on a principle similar to relaxing retinotomy, as a solution for this scenario.

TREATMENT FOR DESCEMET'S MEMBRANE DETACHMENT BASED ON CLASSIFICATION

The treatment of the aforementioned conditions also differs from each other. Although both RDD and TDD require internal gas tamponade or pneumodescemetopexy and sub-Descemet fluid drainage—which is analogous to internal tamponade and subretinal fluid drainage in retinal detachments—TDD also requires relief or removal of the element of traction for the Descemet's membrane to settle onto the stroma. This can be done by relaxing descemetotomy incisions. In the presence of synechiae causing TDD, it may also require synechiolysis and membrane peeling to remove tractional fibrotic bands that pull on the Descemet's membrane. Sub-Descemet fluid drainage is carried out by injecting gas from the side opposite to the tear (internal drainage) or, in some cases, by making a small stab incision in the cornea overlying the Descemet's membrane detachment to drain the fluid externally.

Relaxing descemetotomy may be performed with the anterior chamber filled with viscoelastic or air. The tip of a 26-gauge needle is bent in the reverse direction, as in a capsulotomy needle, and is introduced into the anterior chamber to make the relaxing descemetotomy incisions (Figure 16-3). The extent of the incision is determined during surgery by assessing the degree of foreshortening that still remains. If foreshortening is not completely relieved, the incisions are further extended until the Descemet's membrane is able to lie fully apposed against the stroma. These incisions are made in the peripheral cornea, thereby avoiding the pupillary plane and the visual axis. Postoperative tamponade with nonexpansile concentration of C3F8 (14%) or SF6 (12%) is administered with face-up positioning of the patient for 1 hour (Figure 16-4). A reattachment may not occur in all cases, depending on the extent of inflammatory fibrotic damage to the endothelium, in which case the patient may require a posterior lamellar or full-thickness graft.

Figure 16-3. Relaxing descemetotomy is done to relieve the tension and stress forces acting on the TDD. Once the relaxing descemetotomy cuts are made (arrows), the Descemet's membrane becomes lax and can now be apposed to the overlying corneal stroma by injecting an air bubble.

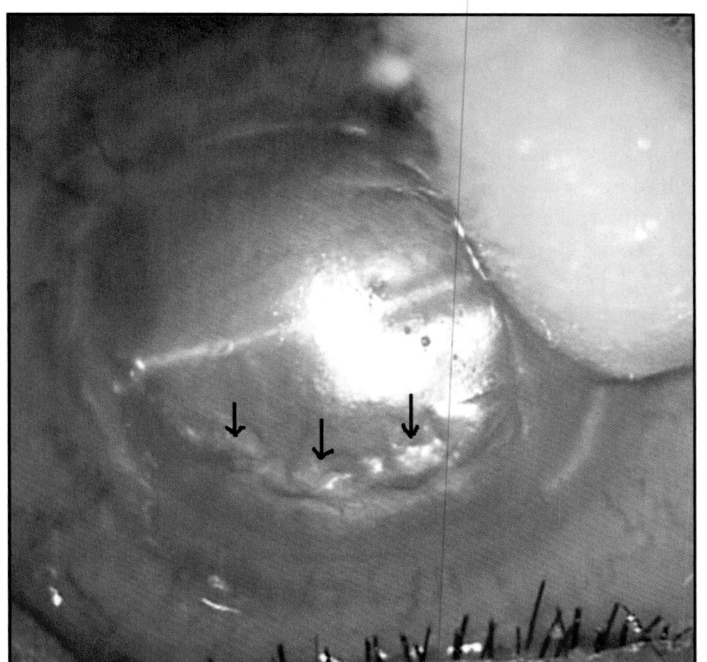

Figure 16-4. (A) Preoperative OCT shows a TDD. (B) Postoperative OCT shows the Descemet's membrane attached after relaxing descemetotomy was performed. (Reprinted with permission from Agarwal A, Jacob S. Relaxing descemetotomy relieves stress forces in taut Descemet's membrane detachment. *Ocular Surgery News.* October 10, 2010:113.)

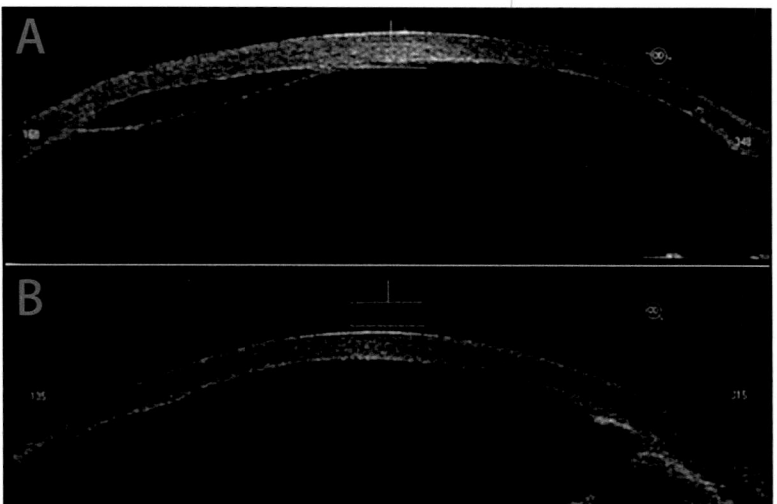

The term *descemetotomy* was first used by Lowenstein in 1993.[21-24] It was used with reference to a procedure where the neodymium-doped yttrium aluminum garnet (Nd:YAG) laser was used in the postoperative period to perform descemetotomy in order to create communication between the anterior chamber and the supernumerary chamber after intentionally retaining the DM during keratoplasty for bullous keratopathy. The authors of those studies found that the membrane was resistant to Nd:YAG laser and required the use of high-energy levels and multiple pulses. Steinemann et al[25] and Masket et al[26] also used the Nd:YAG laser to create a central opening in inadvertently retained opacified host Descemet's membrane after penetrating keratoplasty. Chen et al[27] surgically removed a similarly retained host Descemet's membrane after keratoplasty.

The authors had previously used the term *iatrogenic descemetorhexis*[14] for a case where accidental descemetorhexis occurred in a patient during phacoemulsification. A similar case was also reported by Pan and Au Eong.[15] Descemetorhexis has been described as part of endothelial keratoplasty procedures, where the central Descemet's membrane is intentionally removed from the host cornea.[28-32] The term *relaxing descemetotomy*, which the authors have coined, differs from the aforementioned terms in that it describes a therapeutic procedure that relieves the traction forces and decreases foreshortening of the Descemet's membrane in a procedure similar to that of relaxing retinotomy. The relaxing descemetotomy incisions break the stress forces acting on the Descemet's membrane. The tautness of the Descemet's membrane is relieved, and an air or gas bubble is able to appose the now lax Descemet's membrane against the overlying corneal stroma. A long-acting gas, such as C3F8 or SF6, may be preferable over an air bubble to provide a longer period of tamponade, such as is sometimes preferred in RDD.[11,12]

INTRAOCULAR LENS IMPLANTATION IN THE PRESENCE OF CORNEAL DAMAGE

The authors prefer to use the glued IOL technique with Descemet stripping automated endothelial keratoplasty (DSAEK) in cases with aphakic corneal decompensation. The authors have also used it in cases requiring full-thickness keratoplasty, as well as DMEK. It is important to make the anterior segment stable if combining posterior lamellar keratoplasty techniques with glued IOL implantation. A pupilloplasty may be required for widely dilated, nonconstricting pupils to attain a good air fill in the anterior chamber at the end of surgery, as well as to avoid donor graft dislocation. Intracameral Miochol-E should be instilled after implanting the glued IOL in order to constrict the pupil. This allows a good compartmentalization of the eye into a bicameral structure allowing a greater support for the donor tissue. In the authors' experience of DSAEK combined with glued IOL implantation, there has been no incidence of donor dislocation into the posterior segment. The authors feel the difference from sutured secondary posterior chamber IOLs lies in the rigid, nonelastic attachment of the IOL to the sclera with the glued IOL technique. The crystalline lens-bag-zonule complex—due to its 360-degree attachment to the ciliary area—is a trampoline-like structure (Figure 16-5). However, the Prolene sutures (2 or 4, depending on the technique) used for suture fixating an IOL to the sclera act as a hammock, which provides less torsional stability than the natural state. The glued IOL reduces the torsional and oscillatory freedom of the implant because the resultant IOL-haptic-sclera complex is more stable than the IOL-haptic-suture-sclera complex of the suture-fixated IOLs. This same biomechanical model is the reason for less pseudophakodonesis seen after glued IOL compared to suture-fixated IOL. The learning curve for the glued IOL procedure is fairly simple for most anterior segment surgeons, and the detailed steps for the combination surgery have been provided earlier in the literature as well as in this book. Other authors also noted the disastrous complications of the donor lenticule falling into the vitreous in aphakic eyes.[34] The placement of a glued IOL in situ before placement of the lenticule compartmentalizes the aphakic eye from a unicameral to bicameral environment. This will produce less instability in the anterior segment and will also act as a rigid barrier to prevent the donor lenticule from falling into the vitreous.

DESCEMET'S MEMBRANE ENDOTHELIAL KERATOPLASTY WITH GLUED INTRAOCULAR LENSES

DMEK has been described by Melles[35] for pseudophakic bullous keratopathy (Figure 16-6A). The basic technique consists of preparing the donor graft by partially trephining it and using a Sinskey hook (Appasamy Associates, Chennai, India) to lift up the edge of the cut Descemet's

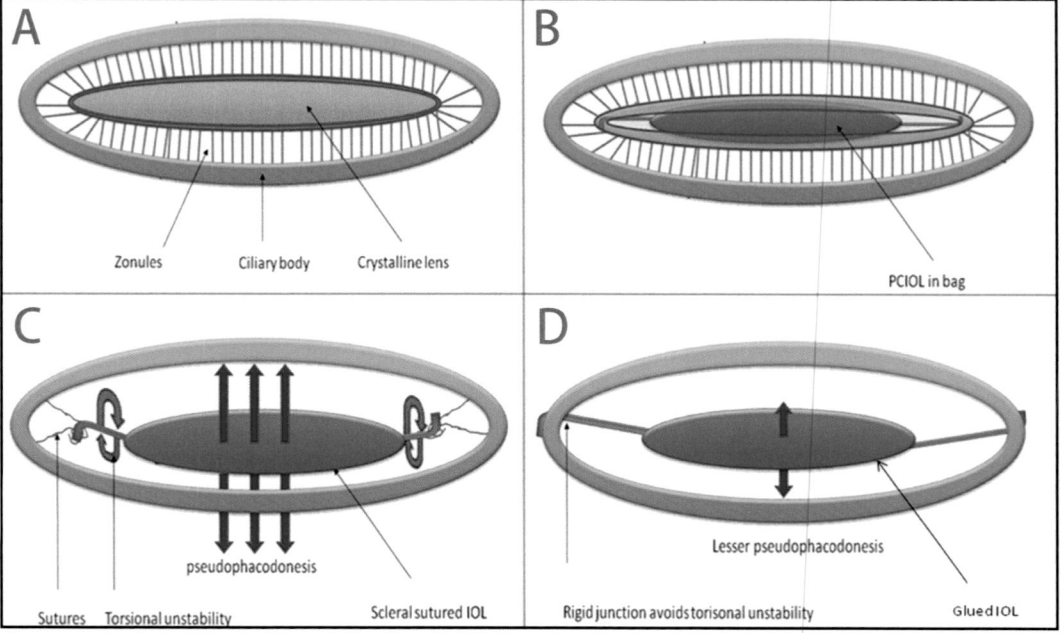

Figure 16-5. IOL implantation and posterior capsular rupture. (A) Schematic diagram showing normal trampoline line arrangement of the ciliary body, zonules, and crystalline lens in a normal eye. (B) Schematic diagram showing the change in the case of a pseudophakic eye with an in-the-bag posterior chamber IOL. (C) Schematic diagram showing a pseudophakic eye with a sutured scleral-fixated IOL with increased torsional instability and increased pseudophakodonesis due to sclera-suture-haptic-optic attachment. (D) Schematic diagram showing a pseudophakic eye with a glued IOL and reduced torsional instability and lesser pseudophakodonesis due to rigid sclera-haptic-optic attachment.

membrane. After an adequate edge is lifted, nontoothed forceps are used to gently grab the Descemet's membrane at its very edge, and the graft is separated from the underlying stroma in a capsulorrhexis-like circumferential manner (Figure 16-6B). These steps are performed using the SCUBA technique described by Gimbel.[36] The DMEK graft is then stained with trypan blue and replaced in the sterile corneal storage medium while the recipient eye is prepared.

An anterior chamber maintainer is inserted and 2 points are marked on the sclera exactly 180 degrees apart. Two 2.5 × 2.5-mm lamellar scleral flaps are created on either side, centered on the marks. Trypan blue is used to stain the patient's Descemet's membrane before scoring and stripping it from approximately 8.5-mm diameter (as marked from above the corneal surface) using a reverse Sinskey hook. A 20-gauge needle is used to create a sclerotomy approximately 1 to 1.5 mm from the limbus under each scleral flap, and a 23-gauge vitrector introduced through the sclerotomy performs anterior vitrectomy. If a posterior chamber IOL is in the anterior chamber, it is repositioned in a closed-globe manner by exteriorizing its haptics through the sclerotomies (Figure 16-7A and 16-7B). If there is an anterior chamber IOL, it is explanted and a new IOL is implanted by performing the conventional glued IOL technique. In aphakic eyes, a foldable IOL is injected into the anterior chamber and its haptics are exteriorized through the sclerotomy. In all situations, once both haptics are exteriorized, the Scharioth tuck is used to tuck them into scleral tunnels made at the edge of the scleral flaps using a 26-gauge needle. Intracameral pilocarpine is then used to constrict the pupil and, if necessary, a pupilloplasty is performed. The graft is then carefully loaded into a Visian implantable contact lens injector (STAAR Surgical, Monrovia, CA), with the cartridge tip held occluded with a finger. It is then injected gently into the anterior chamber by plunging the soft-tipped injector, taking care not to fold the graft (Figure 16-7C). Wound-assisted implantation is avoided, and the anterior chamber maintainer flow is titrated

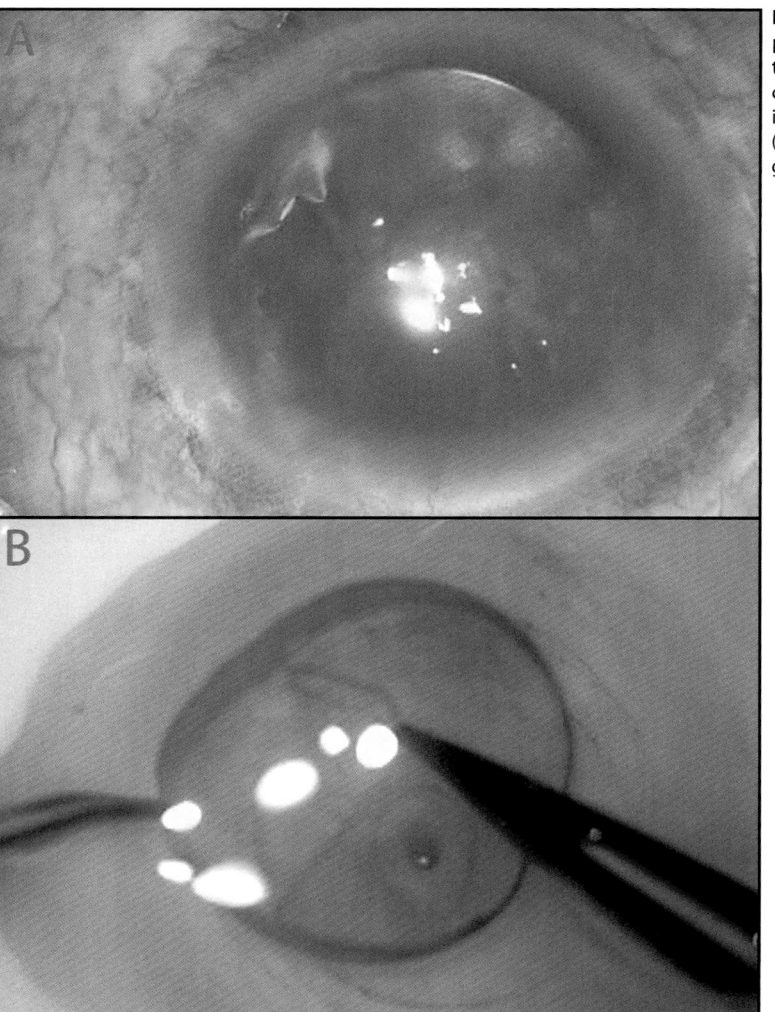

Figure 16-6. (A) Preoperative pseudophakic bullous keratopathy. Note the posterior chamber IOL is implanted in the anterior chamber. (B) Preparation of a DMEK graft.

carefully to prevent backflow and extrusion of the graft through the incision. The graft orientation is then checked and the graft is gently unfolded. Once unfolded, an adequately tight air bubble is injected under the graft to float it up against the stroma (Figure 16-7D). Finally, fibrin glue is used to seal the lamellar scleral flaps, conjunctiva, and the clear corneal incisions.

In patients with aphakia, loss of bicamerality of the eye because of the absence of an iris–lens diaphragm is seen. This leads to poor tamponade effect and posterior migration of the injected air. A disastrous complication can be dislocation of the lenticule into the vitreous cavity. These problems are solved when combining endothelial keratoplasty with a glued IOL.

This technique (endothelial keratoplasty with glued IOL) combines the advantages of stable fixation of the IOL as well as the advantages of lamellar keratoplasty. In contrast, an anterior chamber IOL has the disadvantage of decreased IOL-endothelial distance, which can cause long-term graft failure when combined with penetrating keratoplasty. It becomes especially disadvantageous when combined with DSAEK, where the endothelium with donor stroma also occupies space within the anterior chamber, thereby bringing the anterior surface of the anterior chamber IOL very close to the DSEK lenticule. Hence, these patients require explantation of the anterior chamber IOL, with secondary IOL fixation and corneal transplantation.

Figure 16-7. DMEK with glued IOL. (A) A posterior chamber IOL implanted in the anterior chamber, leading to corneal decompensation. The same posterior chamber IOL is being relocated into the posterior chamber using a closed-globe, glued IOL technique. The haptic is grabbed from over the iris using end-gripping forceps and, using a handshake technique, are transferred between the 2 hands until the tip of the haptic is held. (B) The haptic is exteriorized through the sclerotomy made under the scleral flap. The same procedure is followed for the second haptic, which is exteriorized through a sclerotomy under a second scleral flap created 180 degrees away from the first. Each haptic is then tucked into a scleral tunnel created at the edge of the scleral flap. (C) The DMEK graft is loaded into a Visian implantable contact lens injector and is injected into the anterior chamber.

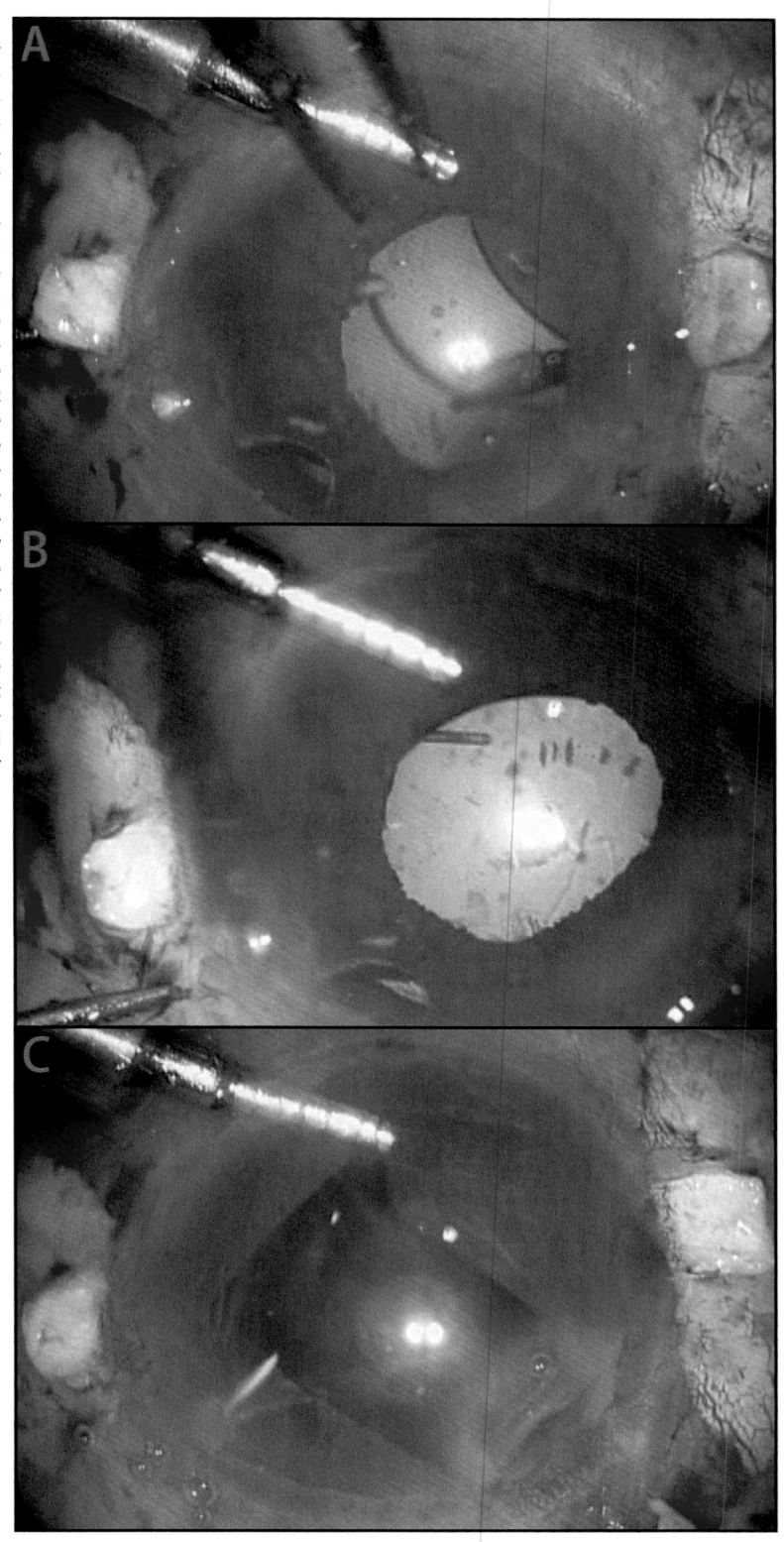

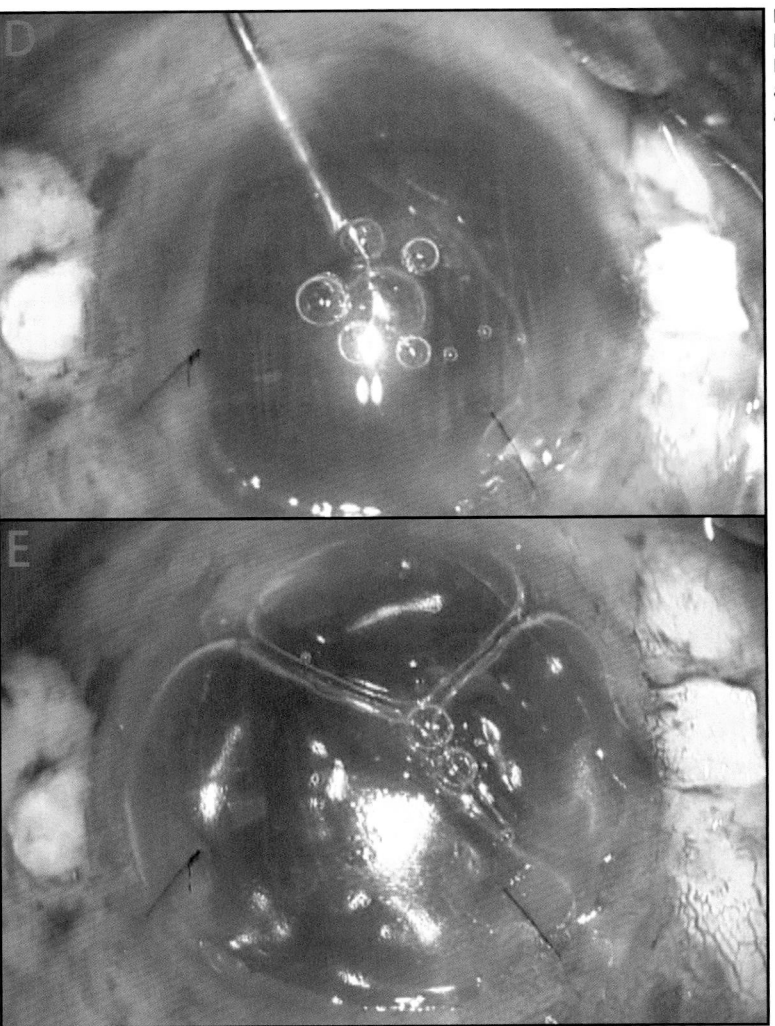

Figure 16-7 (continued). DMEK with glued IOL. (D) The DMEK graft is unrolled. (E) An air bubble is used to appose it against the overlying stroma.

Sutured scleral-fixated IOLs can be combined with endothelial keratoplasty, but it has the disadvantage of a longer open-sky period which makes the patient more vulnerable to potential complications such as expulsive hemorrhage. There is also more pseudophakodonesis associated with sutured IOLs, as the fixation to the sclera is via sutures at 2 points. In the glued IOL technique, the haptic of the IOL itself is anchored to the sclera along a significant portion of its length. This stability of the glued IOL can, in the authors' opinion, lead to a decreased rate of graft dislocation compared to a sutured scleral-fixated IOL, which has more intraocular mobility. The glued IOL also offers the ability to adjust the centration of the IOL at any time during surgery by simply adjusting the degree of tuck of the haptics into the scleral tunnel, unlike the longer and more tedious procedure that would be required to recenter a decentered sutured scleral-fixated IOL. All suture-related complications, such as erosion, degradation, and exposure, are also done away with. The fibrin glue seals the flaps hermetically over the haptics and makes the procedure safe.

REFERENCES

1. Machemer R. Cutting of the retina: a means of therapy for retinal reattachment. *Klin Monbl Augenheilkd.* 1979;175(50):597-601.
2. Machemer R. Retinotomy. *Am J Ophthalmol.* 1981;768-774.
3. Machemer R, McCuen BW, de Juan E. Relaxing retinotomies and retinectomies. *Am J Ophthalmol.* 1986;102:7-12.
4. Alturki WA, Peyman GA, Paris CL, Blinder KJ, Desai UR, Nelson NC. Posterior relaxing retinotomies (analysis of anatomic and visual results). *Ophthalmic Surg.* 1992;23:685-688.
5. Bovey EH, de Juan E, Gonvers M. Retinotomies of 180 degrees or more. *Retina.* 1995;15:394-398.
6. Samuels B. Detachment of Descemet's membrane. *Trans Am Ophthalmol Soc.* 1928;26:427-437. www.ncbi.nlm.nih.gov/pmc/articles/pmx1316706/pdf/taos00073-0462.pdf. Accessed November 15, 2011.
7. Mackool RJ, Holtz SJ. Descemet membrane detachment. *Arch Ophthalmol.* 1977;95:459-463.
8. Kim T, Sorenson A. Bilateral Descemet membrane detachments. *Arch Ophthalmol.* 2000;118:1302-1303.
9. Minkovitz JB, Schrenk LC, Pepose JS. Spontaneous resolution of an extensive detachment of Descemet membrane following phacoemulsification. *Arch Ophthalmol.* 1994;112:551-552.
10. Hoover DL, Giangiacomo J, Benson RL. Descemet membrane detachment by sodium hyaluronate. *Arch Ophthalmol.* 1985;103:805-808.
11. Zusman NB, Waring GO III, Najarian LV, Wilson LA. Sulfur hexafluoride gas in the repair of intractable Descemet's membrane detachment. *Am J Ophthalmol.* 1987;104:660-662.
12. Kim T, Hasan SA. A new technique for repairing Descemet membrane detachments using intracameral gas injection. *Arch Ophthalmol.* 2002;120:181-183.
13. Amaral CE, Palay DA. Technique for repair of Descemet's membrane detachment. *Am J Ophthalmol.* 1999;127:88-90.
14. Agarwal A, Jacob S, Agarwal A, Agarwal S, Kumar MA. Iatrogenic descemetorrhexis as a complication of phacoemulsification. *J Cataract Refract Surg.* 2006;32(5):895-897.
15. Pan JC, Au Eong KG. Spontaneous resolution of corneal oedema after inadvertent 'descemetorhexis' during cataract surgery. *Clin Experiment Ophthalmol.* 2006;34(9):896-897.
16. Dirisamer M, Dapena I, Ham L, et al. Patterns of corneal endothelialization and corneal clearance after Descemet membrane endothelial keratoplasty for Fuchs endothelial dystrophy. *Am J Ophthalmol.* 2011;152(4):543-555.e1.
17. Jacobi C, Zhivov A, Korbmacher J, et al. Evidence of endothelial cell migration after Descemet membrane endothelial keratoplasty. *Am J Ophthalmol.* 2011;152(4):537-542.e2.
18. Balachandran C, Ham L, Verschoor CA, Ong TS, van der Wees J, Melles GRJ. Spontaneous corneal clearance despite graft detachment in Descemet membrane endothelial keratoplasty. *Am J Ophthalmol.* 2009;148(2):227-234.
19. Stewart RMK, Hiscott PS, Kaye SB. Endothelial migration and new Descemet membrane after endothelial keratoplasty. *Am J Ophthalmol.* 2010;149(4):683-684.
20. Cursiefen C, Kruse FE. DMEK: Descemet membrane endothelial keratoplasty. *Ophthalmologe.* 2010;107(4):370-376.
21. Lazar M, Loewenstein A, Geyer O. Intentional retention of Descemet's membrane during keratoplasty. *Acta Ophthalomol.* 1991;69:111-112.
22. Loewenstein A, Geyer O, Lazar M. Intentional retention of Descemet's membrane in keratoplasty for the surgical treatment of bullous keratopathy. *Acta Ophthalmol.* 1993;71:280-282.
23. Loewenstein A, Lazar M. Deep lamellar keratoplasty in the treatment of bullous keratopathy. *Br J Ophthalmol.* 1993;77:538.
24. Loewenstein A, Geyer O, Lazar M. Descemetotomy. *J Cataract Refract Surg.* 1996;22(6):652.
25. Steinemann TL, Henry K, Brown MF. Nd:YAG laser treatment of retained Descemet's membrane after penetrating keratoplasty. *Ophthalmic Surg.* 1995;26(1):80-81.
26. Masket S, Tennen DG. Neodymium:YAG laser optical opening for retained Descemet's membrane after penetrating keratoplasty. *J Cataract Refract Surg.* 1996;22(1):139-141.
27. Chen YP, Lai PC, Chen PY, Lin KK, Hsiao CH. Retained Descemet's membrane after penetrating keratoplasty. *J Cataract Refract Surg.* 2003;29(9):1842-1844.
28. Dapena I, Ham L, Moutsouris K, Melles GR. Incidence of recipient Descemet membrane remnants at the donor-to-stromal interface after descemetorhexis in endothelial keratoplasty. *Br J Ophthalmol.* 2010;94(12):1689-1690.
29. Mehta JS, Hantera MM, Tan DT. Modified air-assisted descemetorhexis for Descemet-stripping automated endothelial keratoplasty. *J Cataract Refract Surg.* 2008;34(6):889-891.

30. Wylegała E, Tarnawska D, Dobrowolski D, Janiszewska D. Outcomes of endothelial keratoplasty with descemetorhexis (DSEK). *Klin Oczna*. 2007;109(7-9):287-291.
31. John T, Bradley JC, McCartney DL, Busin M. Donor corneal disk insertion techniques in descemetorhexis with endokeratoplasty. *Ann Ophthalmol (Skokie)*. 2007;39(4):277-283.
32. Nieuwendaal CP, Lapid-Gortzak R, van der Meulen IJ, Melles GJ. Posterior lamellar keratoplasty using descemetorhexis and organ-cultured donor corneal tissue (Melles technique). *Cornea*. 2006;25(8):933-936.
33. Javadi MA, Feizi S. Deep anterior lamellar keratoplasty using the big-bubble technique for keratectasia after laser in situ keratomileusis. *J Cataract Refract Surg*. 2010;36(7):1156-1160.
34. Singh A, Gupta A, Stewart JM. Posterior dislocation of descemet stripping automated endothelial keratoplasty graft can lead to retinal detachment. *Cornea*. 2010;29(11):1284-1286.
35. Melles GR, Ong TS, Ververs B, van der Wees J. Descemet membrane endothelial keratoplasty (DMEK). *Cornea*. 2006;25(8):987-990.
36. SCUBA technique for DMEK donor preparation. www.youtube.com/watch?v=vpToO8PFsvI

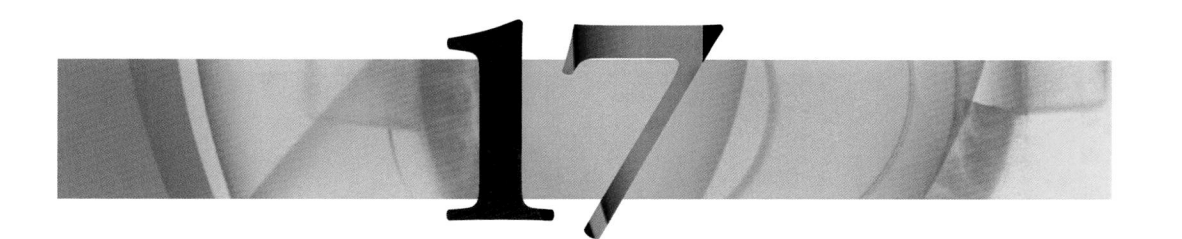

Pseudophakic Cystoid Macular Edema

J. Fernando Arevalo, MD, FACS; Carlos F. Fernandez, MD;
and Fernando A. Arevalo, BS

Cystoid macular edema (CME) following cataract surgery was initially reported by Irvine[1] in 1953 and is known as the Irvine-Gass syndrome.[2] CME is one of the most common causes of unexpected decreased visual acuity after ophthalmic surgery. Despite recent advances in cataract surgery technique and instrumentation, pseudophakic cystoid macular edema (PCME) occurs most frequently after cataract surgery, even after uncomplicated surgery (Figure 17-1).[3] CME exhibits dilation of normal retinal capillaries around the fovea, with consequent fluid leakage and microcystoid formation. It is the pooling of fluorescein in these microcystoid spaces that produces the typical petaloid appearance. CME is often accompanied by disruption of the blood–retinal barrier or blood–aqueous barrier, and, in fact, it is suggested that, clinically, the condition is not limited to the macula, but it spreads and becomes diffuse in the eye.

Although no definitive treatment regimen exists, the long-term goal of treatment is to reduce CME and improve visual acuity.

HISTOLOGY

CME consists of a localized expansion of the retinal intracellular and/or extracellular space in the macular area. This predilection to the macular region is probably associated with the loose binding of inner-connecting fibers in Henle's layer, allowing for the accumulation of fluid leaking from perifoveal capillaries. The absence of Müller cells in the foveal region is also a contributing factor. Radially orientated cystoid spaces consisting of ophthalmoscopically clear fluid are often clinically detectable in the macular area. The cysts are characterized by an altered light reflex with a decreased central reflex and a thin, highly reflective edge. Histological studies show the cysts to be areas of retina in which the cells have been displaced (Figure 17-2).[4] Recently, Antcliff et al[5] monitored the hydraulic conductivity of the human retina following progressive ablation of retinal layers, which is performed with the aid of an excimer laser. They concluded that the inner and

Agarwal A.
Posterior Capsular Rupture: A Practical Guide
to Prevention and Management (pp 199-209).
© 2014 Taylor & Francis Group.

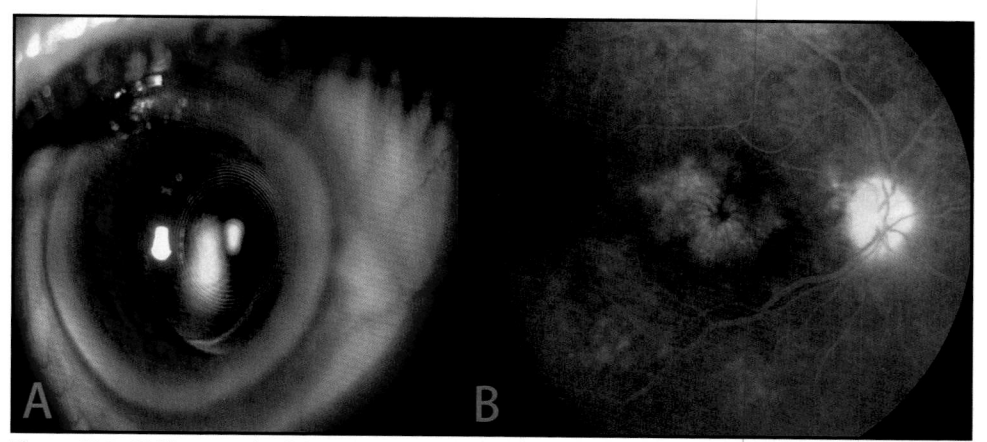

Figure 17-1. (A) Photograph of the anterior segment after uneventful cataract surgery showing a multifocal intraocular lens (IOL) in the posterior chamber. (B) Fluorescein angiography shows pseudophakic CME.

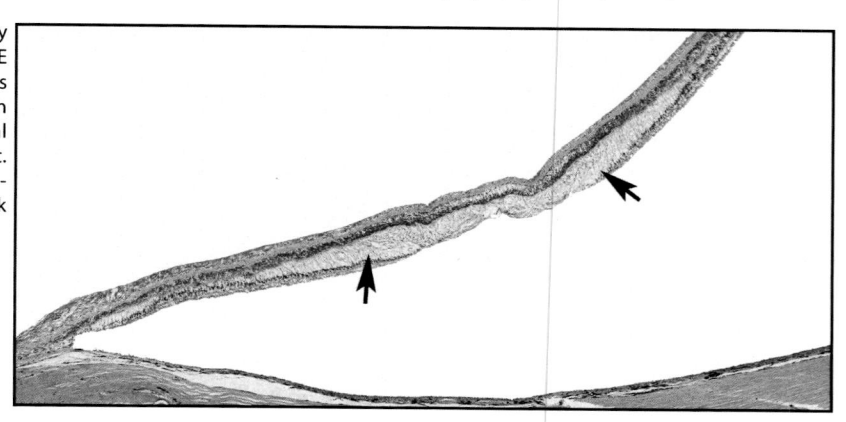

Figure 17-2. Histology of pseudophakic CME showing cystic spaces in the outer plexiform layer (arrows). Retinal detachment is an artifact. (Reprinted with permission from Dr. Deepak Edward.)

outer plexiform layers constitute high-resistance barriers to fluid flow through the retina, which accounts for the characteristic distribution of CME seen in histological specimens and with optical coherence tomography (OCT). In CME associated with cataract extraction, the cysts were most prominent in the inner nuclear layer and less prominent in the outer plexiform layer.

PATHOGENESIS

Several theories exist regarding the pathogenesis of CME,[6,7] and the rationale for its treatment is dictated by the pathogenetic theory. The theories involve changes in the perifoveal retina, where the vascular permeability of the retinal capillaries is altered, leading to leakage of plasma into the central retina which causes it to thicken because of excess interstitial fluid. The excess interstitial fluid is likely to disrupt ion fluxes, and the thickening of the macula results in stretching and distortion of neurons. Reversible reduction in visual acuity occurs, but over time the perturbed neurons die, which results in permanent visual loss (Figure 17-3).[8-13]

The macular region, by virtue of its anatomic structure, is the site of predilection for the accumulation of interstitial fluid. Here, the long neural receptor cell axons radiating outward from the foveal area form the outer plexiform layer of Henle, which acts much like a sponge in that it

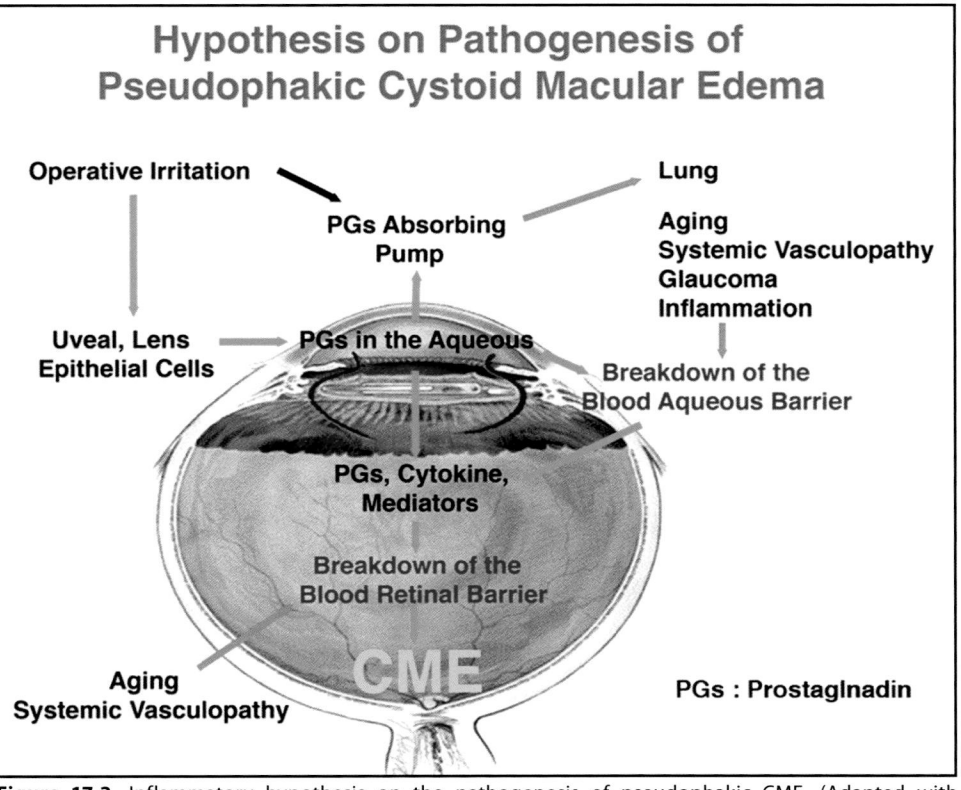

Figure 17-3. Inflammatory hypothesis on the pathogenesis of pseudophakic CME. (Adapted with permission from Miyake K, Ibaraki N. Prostaglandins and cystoid macular edema. *Surv Ophthalmol.* 2002;47[suppl 1]:S203-S218.)

is capable of interstitial accumulation of large quantities of fluid exuding from the neighboring capillaries. As this fluid dissects into the nerve fiber layer, it displaces the nerve fibers to form large lakes of intercellular fluid. Larger lakes develop centrally as a result of the longer nerve fiber layers that are present centrally in Henle's fiber layer.

Fluorescein angiograms often show that the capillaries in the macular region (and disk) are preferentially affected. They show obvious dye leakage, whereas capillaries in other parts of the retina do not. Thus, there is something about these capillaries, or their relation to the vitreous, that makes them preferentially susceptible. The explanation for this preferential increased permeability of the macular capillaries is unknown. All treatment schemes have been related to theoretical factors believed to be associated with its pathogenesis. These include hypotony, hyaluronidase in the local anesthetic, topical adrenergic compounds, phototoxicity induced by the coaxial illumination of the operating microscope, vitreomacular traction, inflammation of macular capillaries potentiated or produced by mediators such as prostaglandins, and the specifics of the cataract technique.

Cataract surgery in diabetic patients may result in a dramatic acceleration of preexisting diabetic macular edema, leading to poor functional visual outcome (Figure 17-4). This can be prevented, provided the severity of the retinopathy is recognized preoperatively and treated appropriately with prompt laser photocoagulation either before surgery, if there is adequate fundal view, or shortly afterward.

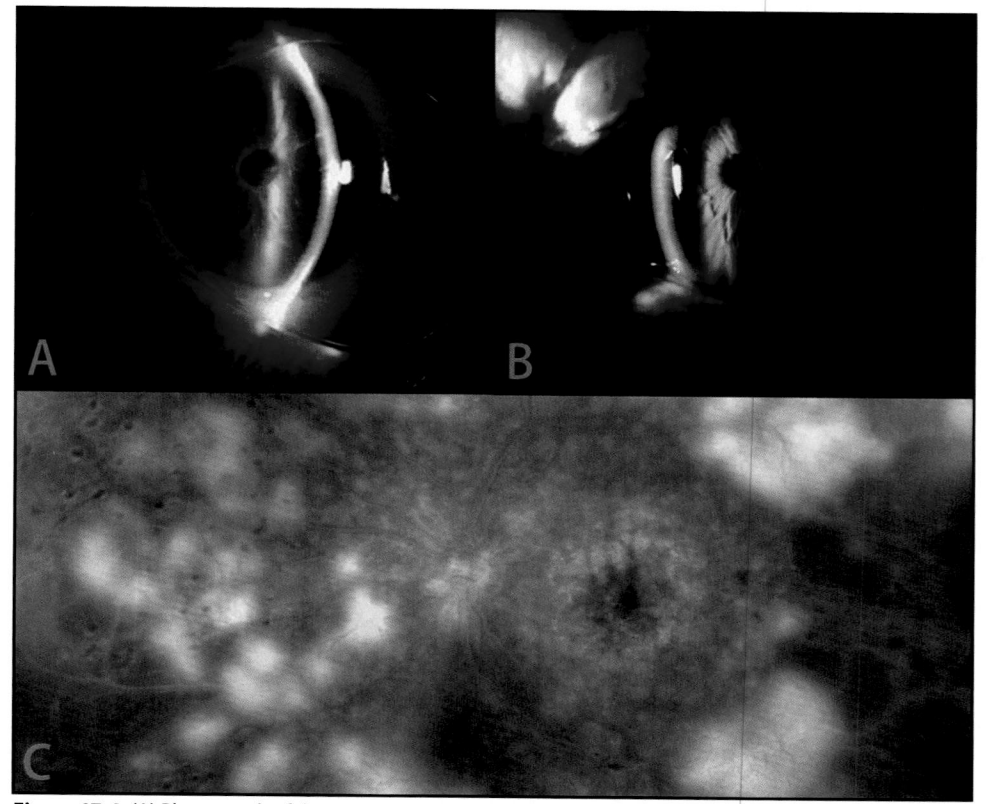

Figure 17-4. (A) Photograph of the anterior segment after uneventful phacoemulsification cataract surgery showing anterior chamber fibrin in a patient with diabetes. (B) Photograph of the anterior segment post-treatment with tissue plasminogen activator (tPA) in the anterior chamber showing disappearance of the fibrin. (C) Fluorescein angiography after cataract surgery showing macular edema and proliferative diabetic retinopathy.

NATURAL HISTORY

Approximately 20% of patients who undergo uncomplicated phacoemulsification or extracapsular extraction develop angiographically proven CME. However, a clinically significant decrease in visual acuity is seen only in approximately 1% of these eyes. If cataract extraction is complicated by posterior capsular rupture and vitreous loss, severe iris trauma, or vitreous traction at the wound, there is a significantly higher incidence (up to 20%) of clinically apparent CME, which is unrelated to the presence of an anterior chamber IOL. Clinically significant CME usually occurs within 3 to 12 weeks postoperatively, but in some instances, its onset may be delayed for months or years after surgery. Spontaneous resolution of CME with subsequent visual improvement may occur within 3 to 12 months in 80% of patients. Chronic CME is defined as a persistent decline in visual acuity for more than 6 months. The longer the CME persists, the less likely it is that the CME will resolve spontaneously. These chronic changes, including the presence of photoreceptor/ retinal pigment epithelium changes or lamellar holes, may result in poor visual acuity even after CME resolves.

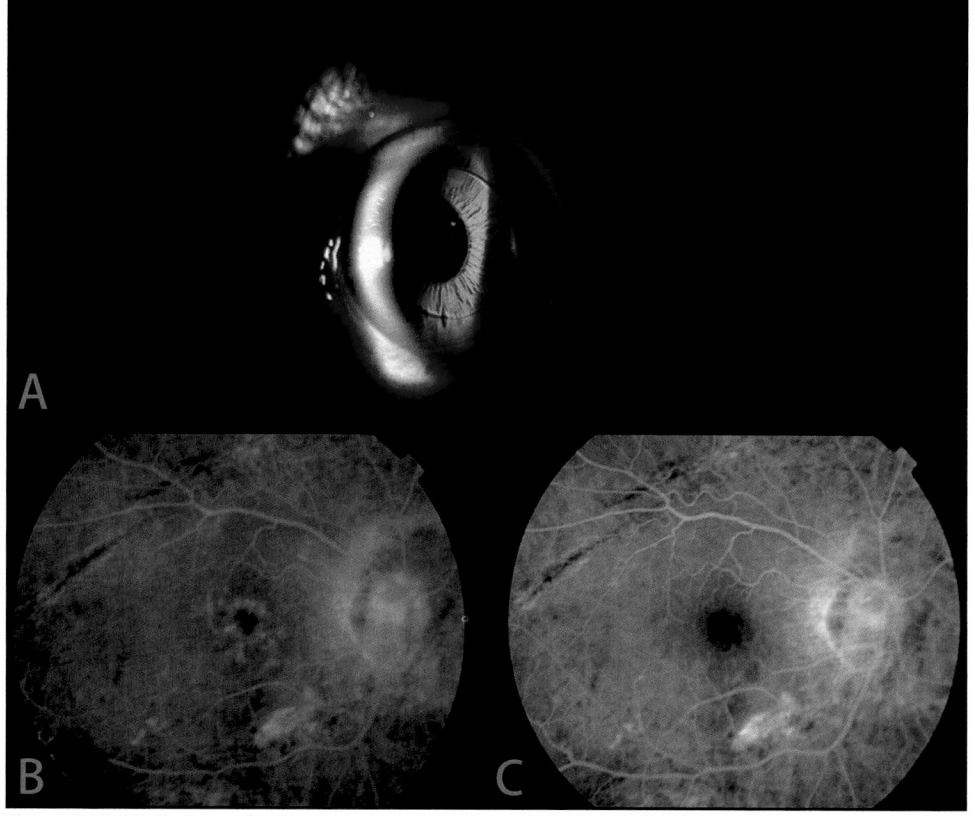

Figure 17-5. (A) Photograph of the anterior segment showing the anterior chamber IOL due to vitreous loss and posterior capsular rupture. (B) Fluorescein angiography showing pseudophakic CME. (C) Fluorescein angiography showing the resolution of the CME after intravitreal bevacizumab.

Interestingly, complicated cataract extraction is associated with an increased risk for clinically significant CME. CME is more often seen in association with some complications of cataract surgery, such as disruption of the anterior vitreous hyaloid (Figure 17-5), vitreous loss, retention of lens cortex, vitreous strands to the wound (Figure 17-6), dislocated IOL, inadequate wound closure, and chronic inflammation.[14]

DIFFERENTIAL DIAGNOSIS

A variety of ocular and systemic diseases can mimic pseudophakic CME and the differential diagnosis can be extensive. Branch retinal vein occlusion or diabetic macular edema can be responsible for the macular edema. Inflammatory diseases can be responsible for macular edema due to the release of inflammatory mediators. Retained lens material may act as a potential source for the release of inflammatory mediators, leading to the development of postoperative CME. Epiretinal membrane formation and vitreomacular traction syndrome are other important causes of mechanical thickening. Finally, the topical use of epinephrine in aphakic patients, prostaglandin analogues, and the use of high doses of nicotinic acid for the treatment of hypercholesterolemia can produce CME.

Figure 17-6. (A) Photograph of the anterior segment showing vitreous strands to the wound. (B) Fluorescein angiography showing CME.

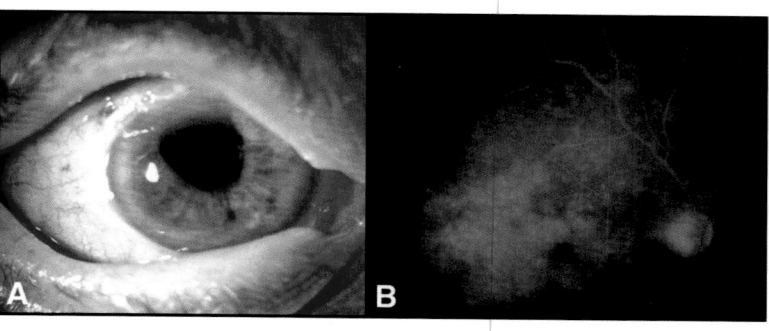

Figure 17-7. Fluorescein angiography showing the classic petaloid appearance in a patient with pseudophakic CME.

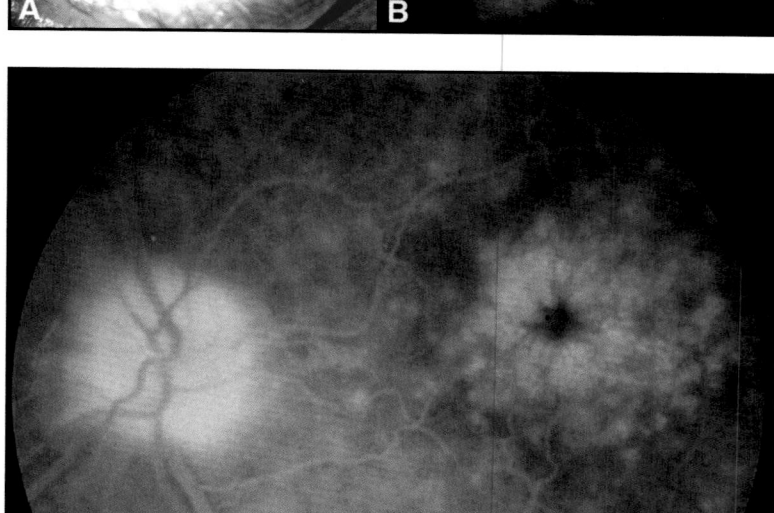

CLINICAL PRESENTATION

Pseudophakic CME should be suspected when a patient without underlying risk factors complains of decreased vision or metamorphopsia following cataract extraction. Clinically, intraretinal edema contained in cyst-like spaces in a honeycomb pattern around the fovea can be seen. A yellow spot in the deep retina replaces the normal foveal reflex. Small intraretinal hemorrhages may sometimes be present within the cystoid spaces. The cystoid spaces may coalesce into a central larger space in chronic edema and a lamellar hole can develop. Diagnosis is based on the clinical findings and its characteristic appearance on fundus fluorescein angiography and OCT.

Angiographic CME is defined as CME that is not clinically noted by the physician or patient and is only detectable with fluorescein angiography. The angiogram is characteristic. Early phases of fluorescein angiography demonstrate dye leakage from the parafoveal retinal capillaries, and later phases of the angiogram demonstrate the petaloid pattern of leakage into the parafoveal intraretinal spaces along with optic disk hyperfluorescence (Figure 17-7).

OCT is a sensitive, noninvasive tool that can clearly show these cystoid spaces as well as calculate central macular thickness and total macular volume. Spectral-domain OCT (SD-OCT), can be used to describe the ultra structural changes. SD-OCT can show an increased thickness of the

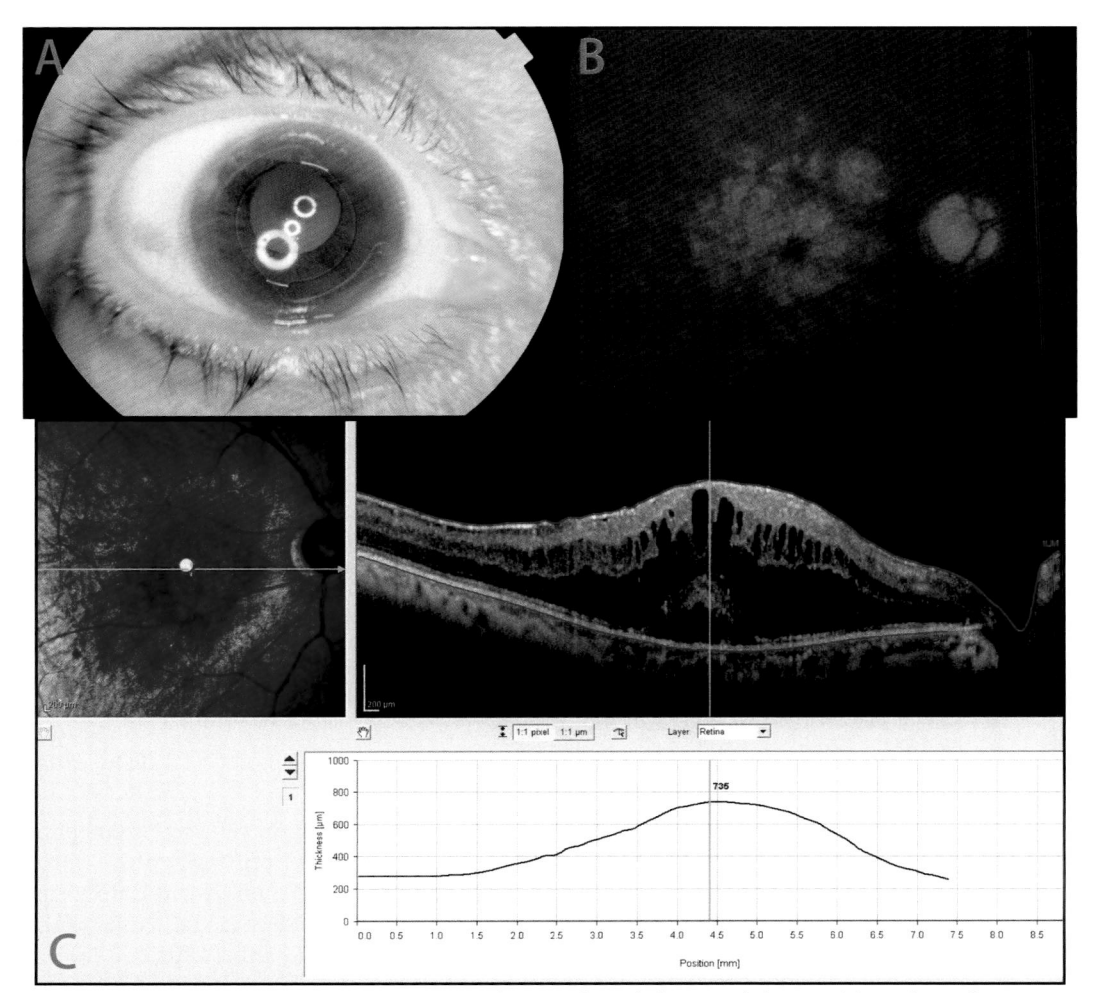

Figure 17-8. (A) Anterior chamber IOL in a patient after complicated phacoemulsification. (B) Late frame fluorescein angiogram demonstrating hyperfluorescence in a petalloid CME pattern in the same patient. (C) SD-OCT can be used to describe the ultra structural changes and show an increased thickness of the fovea and presence of large cystoid spaces in the outer plexiform layer with stretching of the Müller cell processes. In CME associated with cataract extraction, the cysts are most prominent in the inner nuclear layer and less prominent in the outer plexiform layer (left green line represents the site in the retina where horizontal scan was taken, and right vertical line represents where the central retinal thickness [735 μm] is measured).

fovea and the presence of large cystoid spaces in the outer plexiform layer with stretching of the Müller cell processes. OCT can also show increased thickness of the outer-nuclear layer. The photoreceptor layer (as represented by inner segment-outer segment line [IS-OS line]) can be intact, and the continuity of the external limiting membrane can be maintained (Figure 17-8).

PREVENTION

Several trials have evaluated the effect of prophylactic nonsteroidal anti-inflammatory drugs (NSAIDs), and they show that the prophylactic use of NSAIDs reduces the incidence of pseudophakic CME.[15-20] The efficacy of prophylactic nonsteroidal anti-inflammatory therapy is greatest when it is started at least 3 days preoperatively and continued postoperatively for several weeks.

TREATMENT OPTIONS

The primary goal of postsurgical CME treatment is to improve visual acuity by decreasing the amount of macular edema once it has formed. Effective and rational treatment rests on understanding the pathophysiology of the disease process itself.

Nonsteroidal Anti-Inflammatory Agents

NSAIDs are cyclooxygenase inhibitors that work by preventing the synthesis of prostaglandins. Because NSAIDs have no effect on preformed or existing prostaglandin levels, treatment before surgical trauma is essential. Topical ketorolac tromethamine (Acular) demonstrates a sustained beneficial effect on the visual acuity of treated patients who have pseudophakic CME. Newer-generation NSAIDs such as bromfenac sodium (Xibrom) and nepafenac have modifications to their chemical structure which increase ocular penetration and theoretical potency.[21-23]

Nonsteroidal Anti-Inflammatory Drugs Plus Corticosteroids

Several studies have shown the beneficial effect of topical NSAIDS in the prophylaxis and treatment of postoperative CME. Heier et al[24] described a trial that showed the treatment of acute, visually significant pseudophakic CME with a combined therapy of corticosteroid and NSAIDs resulted in greater gains of visual acuity, faster recovery, and greater likelihood of improvement in contrast sensitivity than monotherapy. The combination therapy of topical prednisolone forte 1% 4 times daily plus topical ketorolac 0.5% 4 times daily for 3 months is recommended.

Corticosteroid Injections

Corticosteroids work by inhibiting the release of arachidonic acid from cell membrane phospholipids, thereby preventing the formation of both leukotrienes and prostaglandins. Debate continues regarding the most efficacious route of administration (sub-Tenon's versus intravitreal [IVT]), optimal dosage (4 mg versus greater than 4 mg), and patient safety (as far as the risk of ocular hypertension, retinal detachment, vitreous hemorrhage, and endophthalmitis).

Some studies have demonstrated the usefulness of an IVT injection of triamcinolone acetate in the reduction of pseudophakic CME (Figure 17-9).[25-27]

Carbonic Anhydrase Inhibition

Acetazolamide increases subretinal fluid transport and has been shown to remove foveal cystoid edema in disorders such as retinitis pigmentosa, aphakia, and macular epiretinal membrane formation. However, no patients with primary retinal vascular disorders—such as central retinal vein occlusion or branch retinal vein occlusion—benefited from such treatment. Few case reports correlate the resolution of PCME with use of oral acetazolamide, but, to date, no clinical trials have been performed. Use of acetazolamide is complicated by many potential adverse effects including bone marrow depression, paresthesias, aplastic anemia, gastrointestinal distress, and psychological disturbances.

Anti-Vascular Endothelial Growth Factor Agents

Surgical trauma leads to postoperative inflammation which can ultimately lead to pseudophakic CME through an increase in the production of vasopermeable factors such as vascular endothelial growth factor (VEGF). VEGF has been associated with the breakdown of the blood–retinal

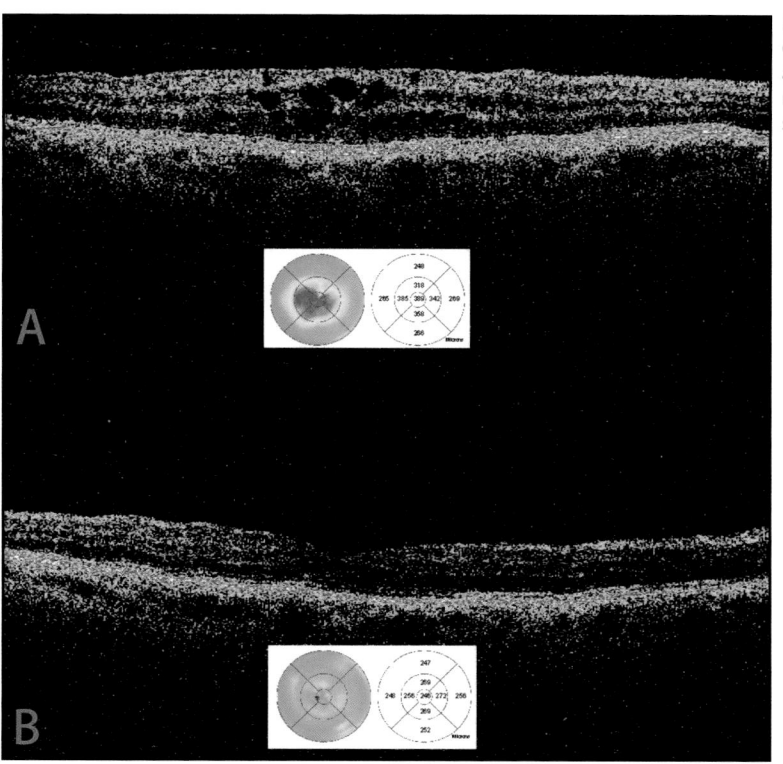

Figure 17-9. (A) Time-domain OCT showing CME. (B) OCT after treatment with intravitreal triamcinolone acetonide showing resolution of CME.

barrier and contributes to the onset of macular edema. VEGF has been demonstrated to increase retinal vessel permeability by increasing the phosphorylation of tight-junction proteins. A recent study showed elevated levels of VEGF and interleukin-6 in ocular fluids of patients with macular edema.[28]

Bevacizumab (Avastin) is a complete, full-length humanized antibody that binds to all subtypes of VEGF-A and is used successfully in tumor therapy as a systemic drug. Recent studies have demonstrated the usefulness of an IVT injection of bevacizumab in the reduction of refractory pseudophakic CME. The mechanism for bevacizumab-induced reduction of CME may be associated with a down regulation of many cytokines and VEGF, combined with conformational changes in the tight junctions of retinal vascular endothelial cells and decrease of vascular permeability.[28-32]

Vitrectomy

Pars plana vitrectomy with membrane peeling may be considered in cases of PCME with a mechanical component that is identified on either clinical examination or by OCT or in cases of chronic refractory edema that is unresponsive to medical therapy.[33,34]

Neodymium-Doped Yttrium Aluminum Garnet Vitreolysis

Pseudophakic CME with vitreous incarceration in the corneoscleral wound responds more slowly than without vitreous incarceration. Some studies report that neodymium-doped yttrium aluminum garnet (Nd:YAG) vitreolysis is effective in the resolution of pseudophakic CME in selected patients with vitreous incarceration.[35,36]

FUTURE DIRECTIONS

As mentioned earlier, corticosteroids work at the beginning of the inflammatory cascade. The dexamethasone intravitreal implant (Ozurdex) is a biodegradable sustained dexamethasone delivery system that is implanted into the vitreous cavity. Its polymer matrix gradually transforms into lactic and glycolic acid, which are, in turn, broken down into water and carbon dioxide. In a Phase II study, 54% of patients experiencing pseudophakic CME and uveitis-associated CME showed an improvement of at least 10 letters of visual acuity at post-implant day 90 compared with only 14% of patients showing a similar result in the observation group (Allergan Phase II study, unpublished data).

Recently, the United States Food and Drug Administration approved triamcinolone acetonide (Triesence) for intravitreal injection during surgery. This drug may be used off-label in the treatment algorithm of recalcitrant pseudophakic CME.

CONCLUSION

Current management of CME includes NSAIDs, NSAIDs plus corticosteroids, corticosteroid injections, carbonic anhydrase inhibition, anti-VEGF agents, vitrectomy, and Nd:YAG vitreolysis. New technology has and will revolutionize the diagnosis, prognosis, and treatment of this condition.

REFERENCES

1. Irvine SR. A newly defined vitreous syndrome following cataract surgery. *Am J Ophthalmol.* 1953;36:599-619.
2. Gass JD, Norton EW. Follow-up study of cystoid macular edema following cataract extraction. *Trans Am Acad Ophthalmol Otolaryngol.* 1969;73:665-682.
3. Wright PL, Wilkinson CP, Balyeat HD, et al. Angiographic cystoid macular edema after posterior chamber lens implantation. *Arch Ophthalmol.* 1988;106:740-744.
4. Tso MO. Pathology of cystoid macular edema. *Ophthalmology.* 1982;89:902-915.
5. Antcliff RJ, Hussain AA, Marshall J. Hydraulic conductivity of fixed retinal tissue after sequential excimer laser ablation: barriers limiting fluid distribution and implications for cystoid macular edema. *Arch Ophthalmol.* 2001;119:539-544.
6. Flach AJ. The incidence, pathogenesis and treatment of cystoid macular edema following cataract surgery. *Trans Am Ophthalmol Soc.* 1998;96:557-634.
7. Stark WJ Jr, Maumenee AE, Fagadau W, et al. Cystoid macular edema in pseudophakia. *Surv Ophthalmol.* 1984;28(suppl):442-451.
8. Nguyen QD, Tatlipinar S, Shah SM, et al. Vascular endothelial growth factor is a critical stimulus for diabetic macular edema. *Am J Ophthalmol.* 2006;142:961-969.
9. Foos RY. Posterior vitreous detachment. *Trans Am Acad Ophthalmol Otolaryngol.* 1972;76:480.
10. Miyake K, Ibaraki N. Prostaglandins and cystoid macular edema. *Surv Ophthalmol.* 2002;47(suppl 1):S203-S218.
11. Yannuzzi LA. A perspective on the treatment of aphakic cystoid macular edema. *Surv Ophthalmol.* 1984;28(suppl):540-553.
12. Jampol LM, Sanders DR, Kraff MC. Prophylaxis and therapy of aphakic cystoid macular edema. *Surv Ophthalmol.* 1984;28(suppl):535-539.
13. Foster RE, Lowder CY, Meisler DM, Zakov ZN. Extracapsular cataract extraction and posterior chamber intraocular lens implantation in uveitis patients. *Ophthalmology.* 1992;99:1234-1241.
14. Spaide RF, Yannuzzi LA, Sisco LJ. Chronic cystoid macular edema and predictors of visual acuity. *Ophthalmic Surg.* 1993;24:262.
15. Henderson BA, Kim JY, Ament CS, et al. Clinical pseudophakic cystoid macular edema. Risk factors for development and duration after treatment. *J Cataract Refract Surg.* 2007;33:1550-1558.
16. Yavas GF, Oztürk F, Küsbeci T. Preoperative topical indomethacin to prevent pseudophakic cystoid macular edema. *J Cataract Refract Surg.* 2007;33:804-807.

17. McColgin AZ, Raizman MB. Efficacy of topical Voltaren in reducing the incidence of post operative cystoid macular edema. *Invest Ophthmol Vis Sci.* 1999;40:S289.
18. Wittpenn JR, Silverstein S, Heier J, et al. A randomized, masked comparison of topical ketorolac 0.4 percent plus steroid vs steroid alone in low-risk cataract surgery patients. *Am J Ophthalmol.* 2008;146:554-560.
19. Wolf EJ, Braunstein A, Shih C, et al. Incidence of visually significant pseudophakic macular edema after uneventful phacoemulsification in patients treated with nepafenac. *J Cataract Refract Surg.* 2007;33:1546-1549.
20. Flach AJ, Stegman RC, Graham J, Kruger LP. Prophylaxis of aphakic cystoid macular edema without corticosteroids. A paired-comparison, placebo-controlled double-masked study. *Ophthalmology.* 1990;97:1253-1258.
21. Walsh DA, Moran HW, Shamblee DA, et al. Anti-inflammatory agents 3. Synthesis and pharmacological evaluation of 2-amino-3-benzoylphenylacetic acid and analogues. *J Medicinal Chem.* 1984;27:1379-1388.
22. Waterbury LD, Silliman D, Jolas T. Comparison of cyclooxygenase inhibitory activity and ocular anti-inflammatory effects of ketorolac tromethamine and bromfenac sodium. *Curr Med Res Opin.* 2006;22:1133-1140.
23. Walters TR, Raizman M, Ernest P, et al. In vivo pharmacokinetics and in vitro pharmacodynamics of nepafenac, amfenac, ketorolac, and bromfenac. *J Cataract Refract Surg.* 2007;33:1539-1545.
24. Heier JS, Topping TM, Baumann W, et al. Ketorolac versus prednisolone versus combination therapy in the treatment of acute pseudophakic cystoid macular edema. *Ophthalmology.* 2000;107:2034-2038.
25. Koutsandrea C, Moschos MM, Brouzas D, et al. Intraocular triamcinolone acetonide for pseudophakic cystoid macular edema: optical coherence tomography and multifocal electroretinography study. *Retina.* 2007;27:159-164.
26. Boscia F, Furino C, Dammacco R, et al. Intravitreal triamcinolone acetonide in refractory pseudophakic cystoid macular edema: functional and anatomic results. *Eur J Ophthalmol.* 2005;15:89-95.
27. Karacorlu M, Ozdemir H, Karacorlu S. Intravitreal triamcinolone acetonide for the treatment of chronic pseudophakic cystoid macular oedema. *Acta Ophthalmol Scand.* 2003;81:648-652.
28. Noma H, Minamoto A, Funatsu H, et al. Intravitreal levels of vascular endothelial growth factor and interleukin-6 are correlated with macular edema in branch retinal vein occlusion. *Graefes Arch Clin Exp Ophthalmol.* 2006;244:309-315.
29. Arevalo JF, Garcia-Amaris RA, Roca JA, et al. Primary intravitreal bevacizumab for the management of pseudophakic cystoid macular edema: pilot study of the Pan-American Collaborative Retina Study Group. *J Cataract Refract Surg.* 2007;33:2098-2105.
30. Barone A, Russo V, Prascina F, Delle Noci N. Short-term safety and efficacy of intravitreal bevacizumab for pseudophakic cystoid macular edema. *Retina.* 2009;29:33-37.
31. Spitzer MS, Ziemssen F, Yoeruek E, et al. Efficacy of intravitreal bevacizumab in treating postoperative pseudophakic cystoid macular edema. *J Cataract Refract Surg.* 2008;34:70-75.
32. Arevalo JF, Maia M, Garcia-Amaris RA, et al; and Pan-American Collaborative Retina Study Group. Intravitreal bevacizumab for refractory pseudophakic cystoid macular edema: the Pan-American Collaborative Retina Study Group results. *Ophthalmology.* 2009;116:1481-1487.
33. Pendergast SD, Margherio RR, Williams GA, et al. Vitrectomy for chronic pseudophakic cystoid macular edema. *Am J Ophthalmol.* 1999;128:317-323.
34. Peyman GA, Canakis C, Livir-Rallatos C, et al. The effect of internal limiting membrane peeling on chronic recalcitrant pseudophakic cystoid macular edema: a report of two cases. *Am J Ophthalmol.* 2002;133:571-572.
35. Steinert RF, Puliafito CA. Anterior Vitreolysis and Cystoid Macular Edema. In: *The Nd:YAG Laser in Ophthalmology: Principles and Clinical Applications of Photodisruption.* Steinert RF, Puliafito CA (Eds). Philadelphia, PA: WB Saunders; 1985:115-123.
36. Steinert RF, Wasson PJ. Neodmium:YAG laser anterior vitreolysis for Irvine-Gass cystoid macular edema. *J Cataract Refract Surg.* 1989;15:304-306.

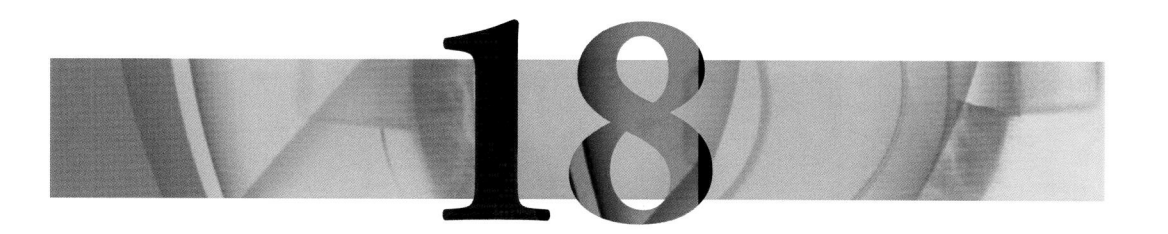

Postoperative Endophthalmitis

Clement K. Chan, MD, FACS

INCIDENCE AND PRESENTATION

The literature has reported the incidence of endophthalmitis[1-40] as ranging from approximately 0.1% to 0.5%.[20] The most common presentation of acute postoperative endophthalmitis includes severe vision loss associated with marked ocular pain and headaches within 2 to 5 days after surgery. However, the Endophthalmitis Vitrectomy Study (EVS)[41] showed that 25% of the patients who developed endophthalmitis in that study lacked pain. The typical ocular findings include a red and painful eye, usually involving lid and corneal edema, chemosis and conjunctival injection and discharge, as well as intraocular infiltrates (ie, hypopyon and vitreous infiltrates) (Figure 18-1).[19] However, the EVS showed that 14% of the patients in that study lacked a hypopyon. In addition, the characteristic clinical signs may be absent or masked due to the application of postoperative antibiotic and corticosteroid drops or an organism with low virulence.

ETIOLOGY

Acute Onset Cases

Gram-positive and coagulase-negative *Staphylococcus* is the most frequent microbial isolate associated with acute postoperative endophthalmitis.

Delayed Onset Cases

Certain cases of postoperative endophthalmitis may have delayed onset. The most common bacterium responsible for delayed-onset and low-grade infection is *Propionibacterium acnes*. Fungal endophthalmitis is another example of delayed-onset infection after surgery.

Agarwal A.
Posterior Capsular Rupture: A Practical Guide
to Prevention and Management (pp 211-220).
© 2014 Taylor & Francis Group.

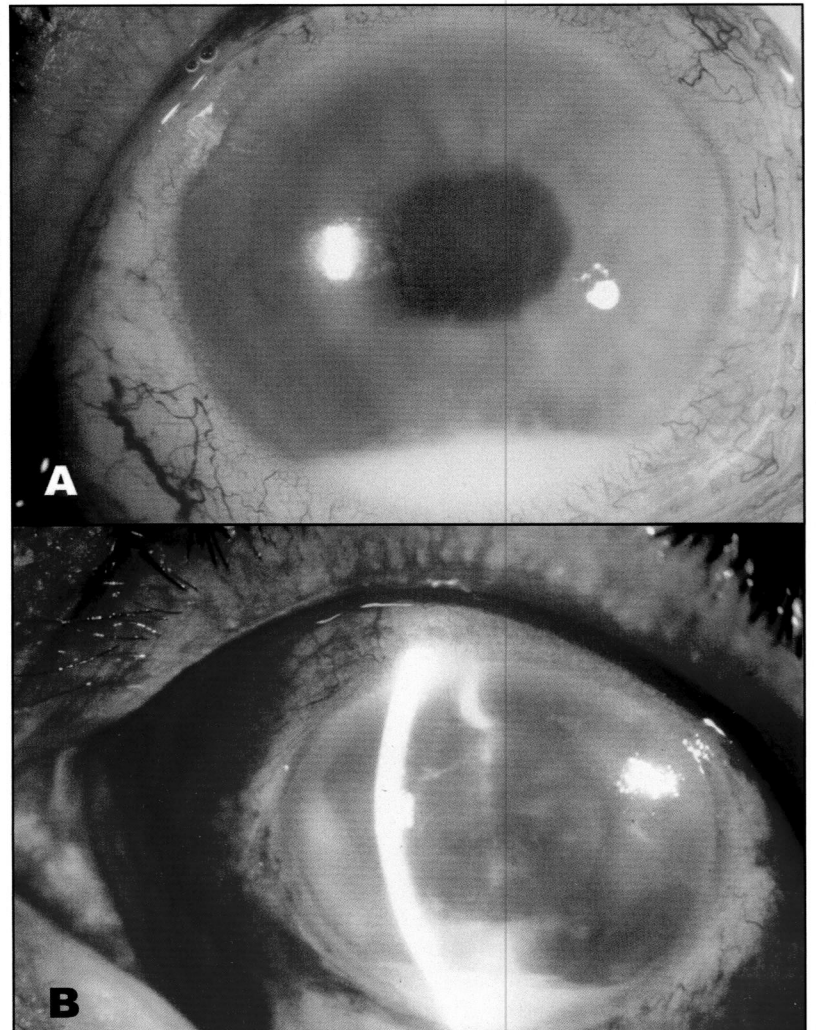

Figure 18-1. Typical examples of acute postoperative endophthalmitis associated with cataract surgery showing the following clinical findings: (A) conjunctival injection hypopyon and (B) vitreous infiltrate. (Reprinted with permission from Chan CC. Postoperative Endophthalmitis. In: Agarwal S, Agarwal A, Agarwal A, ed. *Phacoemulsification.* Jaypee Publishers; 2004:482-497.)

Bleb-Associated Cases

Bleb-associated ocular infection constitutes another distinct category of postoperative ocular infection. The first type involves a less serious and localized form of bleb-related infection which has been given the term *blebitis*[16,21] and includes the conjunctival bleb and the surrounding structures but without vitreous involvement. The second category of bleb-related endophthalmitis is one of the most fulminant forms of ocular infection. For late-onset endophthalmitis, *Streptococcal* species (*S pneumoniae, Enterococcus, Faecalis* [formerly *S faecalis*], *S viridans*, and beta-hemolytic streptococcus) and gram-negative organisms are the most common microbial isolates.

STERILE ENDOPHTHALMITIS

Severe noninfectious intraocular inflammation may develop after surgery in certain eyes. Most of these cases are free of ocular pain, which is an important sign for most cases of infectious endophthalmitis. However, as mentioned previously, the EVS[41] showed that 25% of patients with infectious endophthalmitis may manifest no pain. The sterile inflammation usually starts in the first 24 to 36 hours following surgery, which is somewhat earlier than most incidences of other infections. The clinical findings are also milder than with infectious cases. Conjunctival injection and chemosis may be mild or absent. Anterior chamber reaction may vary from mild to severe. Thus, there may be variable flare and white blood cells, fibrin deposits, and hypopyon. The mild to moderate vitreous infiltrates associated with a sterile endophthalmitis may still allow a residual red reflex from the fundus, in contrast to a severe case of infectious endophthalmitis. Typically, the noninfectious inflammation responds rapidly to steroidal and nonsteroidal medical treatment, without the need for antimicrobial therapy. A high index of suspicion for a missed infection or alternative etiology is needed, if there is a lack of favorable response to anti-inflammatory therapy after 36 to 48 hours. Persistent sterile inflammation may lead to substantial cystoid macular edema (CME) and central visual deficit.

CLINICAL EVALUATION AND DIAGNOSTIC STUDIES

A careful eye examination is required prior to the treatment of the endophthalmitis. The clinician must search for conditions that may be rectified predisposing the patient to endophthalmitis such as iris or vitreous prolapse, wound leak or dehiscence, flat anterior chamber, corneal or suture abscess, bleb defects, and eroding scleral suture associated with a sutured posterior chamber implant. A thorough work-up provides the following advantages for the treating clinician[19]:

- Differentiation of infectious versus sterile endophthalmitis.

- Specific tailoring of the antimicrobial treatment according to the identity and susceptibility of the organism for optimal outcome as a part of the currently accepted practice pattern and medicolegal requirements.

- Creation of sufficient space for delivery of intraocular antimicrobial agents after the vitreous tap. A delay in the specimen collection (particularly after the onset of antimicrobial therapy) may lower the yield of culture-positive results. The standard methods of collecting the aqueous and vitreous specimens may involve a needle tap, a mechanical vitrectomy, or both.

The needle tap method consists of the use of a 30-, 27-, or 25-gauge needle for the collection of 0.1 to 0.25 mL of aqueous specimen, and a 27-, 25-, or larger-gauge needle for the collection of 0.1 to 0.3 mL of a more viscous vitreous specimen. A vitrectomy utilizes a 20-, 23-, or 25-gauge probe with cutting and aspiration functions for collecting up to 0.5 mL of undiluted vitreous specimen through a 1-, 2-, or 3-port approach. For concentration of diluted specimens, either the suction-filtered method or the centrifuged method may yield the optimal outcome (Figure 18-2). The former involves passing a diluted specimen to an upper sterile chamber through a membrane filter with 0.45-micron pores into a lower chamber connected to suction. Using sterile forceps and scissors or knives, the membrane filter containing the concentrated specimen is then cut into small pieces for direct inoculation on solid or liquid media for culturing (Figure 18-2B). Smears may also be prepared from the concentrated specimen. The centrifuged method involves the transfer of the diluted specimen into a sterile centrifuge tube for high-speed centrifuging. The sediments obtained from the centrifuged tube are then processed for microbiological stains and cultures (Figure 18-2C).[19] The most recent advances in diagnostic tools for microbiological work-up for endophthalmitis involve immunologic and molecular genetic technologies that may enhance the speed and specificity of identifying the organisms.

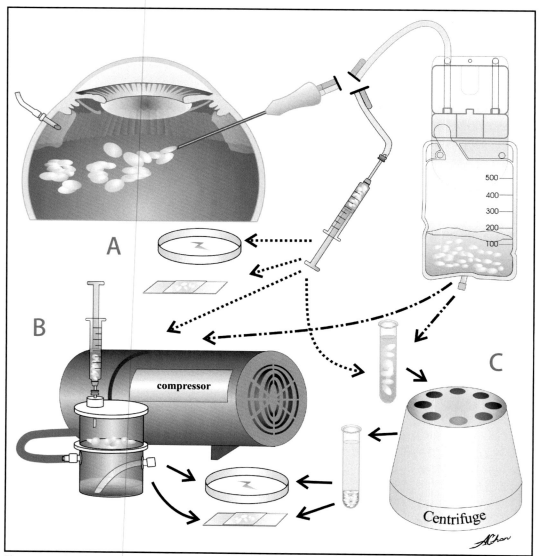

Figure 18-2. (A) The smear preparation and inoculation of culture media can be achieved without further processing for undiluted aqueous and vitreous specimens. A diluted specimen collected in a syringe or vitrectomy cassette needs concentration first via either (B) the vacuum method by passing the diluted fluid in a sterile upper chamber through a 0.45-micron membrane filter into a lower sterile chamber, or (C) the centrifuge method by high-speed centrifuge in a sterile tube. The cut pieces of the membrane filter containing the concentrated specimen or the sediments from the centrifuged tube are then applied on smears for staining and inoculated in culture media for culturing. (Reprinted with permission from CA Chan, Inc.)

PROPHYLACTIC THERAPY

Paying close attention to sterile techniques during surgery and prophylactic antimicrobial treatment constitutes the key measures for preventing postoperative endophthalmitis. Appropriate sterile prepping/draping and the retraction of the eyelids and lashes with a sterile lid speculum are crucial steps in achieving this goal. The application of topical povidone-iodine solution before or during surgery has been shown to be the most effective means of preventing postoperative endophthalmitis.[2]

TREATMENT OF ENDOPHTHALMITIS

Although previous studies have shown the lack of efficacy of topical and subconjunctival antimicrobials after a sufficient quantity of organisms are inoculated into the eye, consistent application of postoperative antimicrobials remains an essential part of effective treatment for postoperative endophthalmitis, particularly for a corneal ulcer, suture or wound abscess, or bleb infection associated with the endophthalmitis.[19,20] Otherwise, topical and subconjunctival therapy constitutes only adjunctive treatment for postoperative endophthalmitis. The standard regimen of topical antibiotic therapy includes the frequent application of broad-spectrum antibiotics that are effective against both gram-positive and gram-negative organisms and the repeated administration of anti-inflammatory corticosteroid and cycloplegic medications. Corticosteroid drops are usually avoided for fungal endophthalmitis. The use of customized, topically fortified antimicrobial therapy for treating postoperative endophthalmitis is a common but controversial practice (eg, 45 to 50 mg/mL of vancomycin, 50 mg/mL of cefazolin, cefamandole, or ceftazidime, 50 mg/mL of ampicillin, 50 mg/mL of clindamycin, 1% solution of methicillin, 8 to 15 mg/mL of tobramycin, 10 to 20 mg/mL of gentamicin or amikacin, 0.15% to 0.5% of amphotericin B, or 10 mg/mL of miconazole).[19] Their superiority over the regular doses of commercially available antimicrobials remains to be unproven. Another frequent but controversial practice is the administration of supplemental subconjunctival antimicrobial injections (eg, 25 mg of vancomycin; 100 to 125 mg of cefazolin or cftazidime; 75 mg of cefamandole; 100 mg of ampicillin or methicillin; 20 to 40 mg of gentamicin, tobramycin, or amikacin; 30 mg of clindamycin, or 5 mg of miconazole). The synergistic effects of subconjunctival and topical antimicrobial therapy combined with intravitreal antimicrobial therapy are unproven.

INTRAVITREAL ANTIMICROBIALS

Currently, the typical empirical antibiotic regimens for intravitreal injections (Table 18-1) include the following:

- Vancomycin (1.0 mg in 0.1 mL of diluent) and ceftazidime (2.25 mg in 0.1 mL)
- Vancomycin (1.0 mg in 0.1 mL of diluent) and amikacin (100 to 400 mcg in 0.1 mL) for beta-lactam sensitive patients

For postoperative fungal endophthalmitis, amphotericin B (5 to 10 mcg per 0.1 mL of diluent) is the drug of choice for intravitreal injections.[4] Because of its potential toxicity, the dosage of amphotericin B needs to be precise.[4] It should also be shielded from light due to its tendency to degrade with light exposure. The alternative is miconazole (25 mcg per 0.1 mL of diluent). Supplemental therapy with subconjunctival miconazole (10 mg in 1 mL) and concurrent intake of oral flucytosine (150 mg/kg/day in 4 divided doses) may provide a synergistic effect with amphotericin B against the fungus. Most recently, intravitreal voriconazole—a new-generation triazole (100 mcg per 0.1 mL of diluent)—has been found to possess high safety and efficacy profiles for treating postoperative and endogenous fungal endophthalmitis.

SYSTEMIC ANTIBIOTICS AND CORTICOSTEROID THERAPY

The EVS[41] determined the lack of further benefits provided by systemic antibiotics in addition to intravitreal antibiotics in treating postoperative endophthalmitis. However, some critics of the EVS have pointed out that the lack of additional benefits of systemic antibiotics might have been due to the limitation in the use of only systemic ceftazidime, ciprofloxacin, and amikacin in the EVS. They contend that had systemic vancomycin and clindamycin been included—as both of

TABLE 18-1. PROTOCOL FOR INTRAVITREAL ANTIBIOTIC PREPARATION

Vancomycin Hydrochloride: 1 mg in 0.1 mL

1. Add 10 mL of diluent to 500 mg powder in a vial, resulting in 50 mg/mL concentration.
2. Insert 2 mL (100 mg) or reconstituted drug into a 10-mL sterile empty vial and add 8 mL of diluent, resulting in a final solution of 10 mg/mL.*

Ceftazidime Hydrochloride: 2.25 mg in 0.1 mL

1. Add 10 mL of diluent to 500 mg powder in a vial, resulting in 50 mg/mL concentration.
2. Insert 1 mL (50 mg) of reconstituted drug into a 10-mL sterile empty vial, and mix with 1.2 mL of diluent for a final solution of 22.5 mg/mL. *

Cefazolin Sodium: 2.25 mg in 0.1 mL

1. Add 2 mL of diluent to 500 mg powder in a vial, resulting in a concentration of 225 mg/mL.
2. Insert 1 mL (22.5 mg) of reconstituted drug into a 10-mL sterile empty vial and mix with an additional 9 mL of diluent for a final solution of 22.5 mg/mL. *

Amikacin Sulfate: 0.2 to 0.4 mg in 0.1 mL

1. Original vial contains 500 mg in 2 mL (250 mg/mL) solution.
2. Add 0.8 mL (200 mg) solution into a 10-mL sterile empty vial and mix with additional 9.2 mL of diluent to achieve a concentration of 200 mg in 10 mL (20 mg/mL).
3. Withdraw 0.2 mL (4 mg) and mix with 0.8 mL of diluent in a second sterile empty vial to achieve final solution of 0.4 mg/mL,* or withdraw 0.1 mL (2 mg) and mix with 0.9 mL of diluent to achieve a final solution of 0.2 mg/mL.*

Gentamicin Sulfate: 0.1 to 0.2 mg in 0.1 mL

1. Original vial contains 80 mg in 2 mL (40 mg/mL) solution.
2. Add 0.1 mL (4 mg) solution into a 10-mL sterile empty vial and mix with 3.9 mL of diluent to achieve a solution of 4 mg in 4 mL or 1 mg/1 mL, * or add 0.2 mL (8 mg) solution into a 10-mL sterile empty vial and mix with 3.9 mL of diluent to achieve a solution of 8 mg in 4 mL or 2 mg/1 mL.*

Clindamycin Phosphate: 1 mg in 0.1 mL

1. Original vial contains a 600 mg in 4 mL solution (15.0 mg/1 mL).
2. Add 0.2 mL (30 mg) solution into a 10-mL sterile empty vial and mix with 2.8 mL of diluent to achieve a solution of 30 mg in 3 mL or 10 mg/mL.*

Chloramphenicol Sodium Succinate: 2 mg in 0.1 mL

1. Original vial contains 1000 mg powder.
2. Add 10 mL of diluent to reconstitute 1000 mg powder for a concentration of 100 mg/mL.
3. Withdraw 1 mL of reconstituted drug (100 mg) and mix with 4 mL of diluent in a 10-mL sterile empty vial to achieve a final solution of 20 mg/1 mL.*

Amphotericin B: 0.005 mg in 0.1 mL

1. Original vial contains 50 mg powder.
2. Add 10 mL of diluent to reconstitute the 50 mg powder into a concentration of 5 mg/mL.
3. Add 0.1 mL (0.5 mg) of reconstituted solution into a 10-mL sterile empty vial and mix with 9.9 mL of diluent to achieve a final solution of 0.05 mg/1 mL.*

Miconazole: 0.025 mg in 0.1 mL

1. Original ampule contains 20 mL of 10 mg/mL solution.
2. Remove glass particles and impurities by passing solution into a 5 micron filter needle.
3. Add 0.25 mL (2.5 mg) of filtered solution into a 10-mL sterile empty vial and mix with 9.75 mL of diluent to achieve a final solution of 2.5 mg in 10 mL, or 0.25 mg/1 mL.

*Single-dose sterile water or bacteriostatic water serves as the diluent.

which are known to be highly effective against gram-positive organisms—the conclusion on the additional value of systemic antibiotics in the EVS might have been different.

A lack of consensus exists regarding intravitreal corticosteroid therapy. Theoretical benefits of corticosteroid therapy include counteractivity against macrophage and neutrophil migration, stabilization of lysosomal membranes, decreased degranulation of inflammatory cells (neutrophils, mast cells, macrophages, and basophils), and reduction in prostaglandin synthesis and capillary permeability due to inhibition of phospholipase A2. However, the harmful effects of corticosteroid therapy include potential reduction in the killing power of inflammatory cells, changes in the bioavailability and doses of the intravitreal antibiotics, potentiation of the infection in the absence of appropriate antibiotic therapy, risk of retinal toxicity due to medication errors, and inability to counteract bacterial toxin-induced damages.

VITRECTOMY FOR TREATING ENDOPHTHALMITIS

Multiple theoretical advantages are associated with vitrectomy for endophthalmitis. For instance, it allows rapid elimination of sequestered infectious infiltrates and vitreous opacities, reduction in inflammatory mediators, relief of vitreoretinal traction, more room for intravitreal injections, and enhanced diffusion of medications.

ENDOPHTHALMITIS VITRECTOMY STUDY

The EVS[11] was a carefully designed, multicenter, controlled prospective clinical trial sponsored by the National Eye Institute. Its definitive conclusions were reported in 1995. The main conclusion of the EVS was for those eyes undergoing cataract extraction with an intraocular implant that developed postoperative endophthalmitis, vitreous tap and intravitreal antibiotic injections alone (TAP) yielded equivalent outcome compared with those eyes treated with immediate vitrectomy and intravitreal antibiotic injections (VIT), (66% versus 62% with final visual acuity of 20/40 or better), as long as the baseline visual acuity was hand motions or better.[11] However, the EVS determined that for those infected eyes with a baseline visual acuity of light perception only, the VIT group fared better than the TAP group.[11] In this latter category, a 3-fold increase in the rate of achieving a visual acuity of 20/40 or better was found in the VIT group compared with the TAP group (33% versus 11%). There was also a 2-fold increase in the rate of achieving a VA of 20/100 and a 50% reduction in the rate of severe visual loss (VA < 5/200) in the VIT group compared with the TAP group (56% versus 30%, and 20% versus 47%, respectively) for these eyes with a baseline VA of hand motions or worse.[11] For the EVS, the designation of achieving a VA of hand motions required the patient to correctly identify 4 of 5 presentations of hand movement shown at 2 feet (60 cm) away, with a light source emanating from behind the patient and directed toward the examiner's hand. Therefore, if the patient could recognize only hand motions at less than 2 feet, the VA would be considered to be light perception only, and a vitrectomy with antibiotic injections would be recommended.

VITRECTOMY TECHNIQUES

Pars plana vitrectomy for postoperative endophthalmitis may utilize a 2- or 3-port, 20-, 23-, or 25-gauge technique. In addition, single-port, 23-gauge vitrectors are now available for simple vitreous biopsy in the office setting (ie, Josephberg 1-port vitrectomy biopsy cutter [Becton Dickinson, Teterboro, NJ] or Intrector [Insight Instruments, Stuart, FL]).

Figure 18-3. Clearance of the anterior chamber before vitrectomy. (A) Anterior chamber washout is used to eliminate cloudy fibrin deposits and hyphema to allow the surgeon to have appropriate visualization before a vitrectomy can be performed. (B) The surgeon may employ a microsurgical pick or hook inserted through the limbus to scrape off the cloudy material from the surfaces of the intraocular lens and iris for removal with a vitrectomy probe. Separate infusion via a cannula connected to a separate infusion line is usually needed through a second limbal incision to prevent the collapse of the anterior chamber during this portion of the procedure. On achievement of appropriate clarity of the anterior chamber, the proper location of the posterior infusion cannula is then ascertained by visualizing its tip before turning on the posterior infusion line. (Reprinted with permission from CA Chan, Inc.)

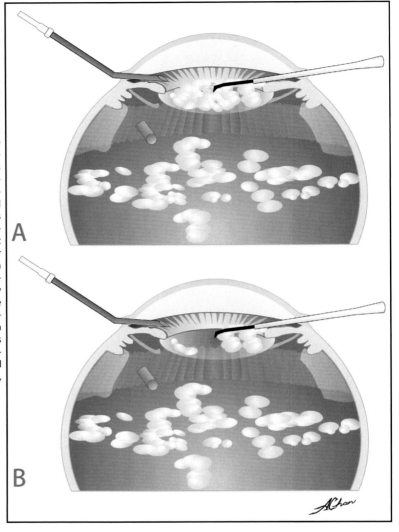

If possible, use a long-infusion cannula (ie, 6 mm) during a vitrectomy, which lowers the risk of inadvertent subretinal and choroidal infusion for pseudophakic eyes with postoperative endophthalmitis, given the multiple predisposing factors of such eyes for surgical complications (eg, limited intraocular tissue visibility, increased choroidal congestion, and frequent hypotony).[19] To further avoid such surgical complications, the surgeon must ensure that the tip of the infusion cannula is well within the vitreous cavity before turning on the infusion fluid. For an eye with very cloudy media, the surgeon may confirm the proper position of the infusion cannula's tip by gently rubbing the tip of a microvitreoretinal (MVR) blade inserted through one of the superior sclerotomies against the tip of the infusion cannula. Frequently, a separate anterior chamber washout through the limbus is required to eliminate cloudy fibrin deposits or hyphema from the anterior chamber first, before attaining sufficient clarify in the anterior portion of the eye for a pars plana vitrectomy.[19] Various microsurgical hooks and picks may be inserted through the limbus to scrape off infiltrates in the anterior chamber and fibrin membranes layered on the surfaces of the implant and the iris before removing them with a vitrectomy probe from the anterior chamber (Figure 18-3). A separate infusion line may be required through the limbus for the anterior chamber wash-out to prevent chamber collapse. When performing a core vitrectomy, care must be taken to engage in only gentle intraocular movements, avoiding vigorous surgical maneuvers that may induce vitreoretinal traction such as aggressive epiretinal membrane removal and fibrin clean-up. Despite the intentional avoidance of their direct removal during the vitrectomy, the posterior epiretinal fibrin deposits and hemorrhage tend to slowly dissolve following injections of intravitreal antimicrobial and anti-inflammatory medications after surgery. To reduce the chance of retinal complications, keep the intraocular instruments well within the anterior and central vitreous cavity and stay away from the fragile infected retina during surgery. The vitreous specimen for microbial investigation is either collected into a syringe connected to the aspiration line of the vitrectomy probe or into a cassette of the vitrectomy machine for subsequent processing (see Figure 18-3). Finally, the eye is made sufficiently soft to allow room for the injection of medications, and the sclerotomies are closed tightly to avoid leakage before injection of intravitreal drugs at the end of the surgery.

CONCLUSION

For the majority of postoperative endophthalmitis that occurs following cataract surgery, relatively favorable visual outcomes can be achieved with prompt and appropriate therapy due to the predominance of coagulase-negative *Staphylococcus* and other low-virulent, gram-positive organisms responsible for the infection. The EVS showed that for those eyes diagnosed with postoperative endophthalmitis following cataract surgery and presenting with visual acuity of hand motions or better, simple vitreous tap and antimicrobial injections alone in the office setting fares as well as immediate vitrectomy and antimicrobial injections.

REFERENCES

1. Forster RK. Endophthalmitis. In: Tasman W and Jaeger EA, eds. *Duane's Clinical Ophthalmology*, Volume 4. Philadelphia, PA: Lippincott-Raven; 1996:1-29.
2. Heilskov T, Joondeph BC, Olsen KR, et al. Case report: late endophthalmitis after transscleral fixation of a posterior chamber intraocular lens. *Arch Ophthalmol.* 1989;107:1427.
3. Christy NE, Lall P. Postoperative endophthalmitis following cataract surgery. *Arch Ophthalmol.* 1973;90:361-366.
4. Kattan HM, Flynn HW Jr, Pflugfelder S, et al. Nosocomial endophthalmitis survey. *Ophthalmology.* 1991;98:227-238.
5. Leveille AS, McMullan FD, Cavanagh HD. Endophthalmitis following penetrating keratoplasty. *Ophthalmology.* 1983;90:38-39.
6. Han DP. Acute-onset postoperative endophthalmitis: current recommendations. In: Syllabus: Subspecialty Day 1998-Retina. Management of posterior segment complications of anterior segment surgery.
7. Starr MB. Prophylactic antibiotics for ophthalmic surgery. *Surv Ophthalmol.* 1983;27:353-373.
8. Javitt JC, Vitale S, Canner JK, et al; National outcomes of cataract extraction. *Arch Ophthalmol.* 1991;109:1085-1089.
9. Wilson FM, Wilson II FM. Postoperataive uveitis. In: Tasman W, Jaeger EA, eds. *Duane's Clinical Ophthalmology,* Volume 4. Philadelphia, PA: Lippincott-Raven; 1996:1-18.
10. Nelson PT, Marcus DA, Bovino JA. Retinal detachment following endophthalmitis. *Ophthalmology.* 1985;92:1112-1117.
11. Endophthalmitis Vitrectomy Study Group. Results of the endophthalmitis vitrectomy study. A randomized trial of immediate vitrectomy and intravenous antibiotics for the treatment of postoperative bacterial endophthalmitis. *Arch Ophthalmol.* 1995;113:1479-1496.
12. Bode DD, Gelender H, Forster RK. A retrospective review of endophthalmitis due to coagulase-negative staphylococci. *Br J Ophthalmol.* 1985;69:915-919.
13. Ormerod LD, Ho DD, Becker LE, et al. Endophthalmitis caused by the coagulase-negative *staphylococci*: I. Disease spectrum and outcome. *Ophthalmology.* 1993;100:715-723.
14. Forster RK, Abbott RL, Gelender H. Management of infectious endophthalmitis. *Ophthalmology.* 1980;87:313-319.

15. Puliafito CA, Baker AS, Haaf J, et al. Infectious endophthalmitis. *Ophthalmology*. 1982;89:921-929.

16. Han DP, Wisniewski SR, Wilson LA, et al. Spectrum and susceptibilities of microbiologic isolates in the Endophthalmitis Vitrectomy Study. *Am J Ophthalmol*. 1996;112:1-17.

17. Theodore FH. Symposium: postoperative endophthalmitis. Etiology and diagnosis of fungal postoperative endophthalmitis. *Ophthalmology*. 1978;85:327-340.

18. Meisler DM, Palestine AG, Vastine DW, et al. Chronic propionibacterium endophthalmitis after cataract extraction and intraocular lens implantation. *Am J Ophthalmol*. 1986;102:733-739.

19. Jaffe GJ, Whitcher JP, Biswell R, et al. Propionibacterium acnes endophthalmitis seven months after extracapsular cataract extraction and intraocular lens implantation. *Ophthalmic Surg*. 1986;17:791-793.

20. Roussel TJ, Culbertson WW, Jaffe NS. Chronic postoperative endophthalmitis associated with Propionibacterium acnes. Arch Ophthalmol. 1987;105:1199-1201.

21. Meisler DM, Zakov ZN, Bruner WE, et al. Endophthalmitis associated with sequestered intraocular Propionibacterium acnes [letter]. *Am J Ophthalmol*. 1987;104:428-429.

22. Brady SE, Cohen EJ, Fischer DH. Diagnosis and treatment of chronic postoperative bacterial endophthalmitis. *Ophthalmic Surg*. 1988;19:580-584.

23. Meisler DM, Mandelbaum S. Propionibacterium-associated endophthalmitis after extracapsular cataract extraction. Review of reported cases. *Ophthalmology*. 1989;96:54-61.

24. Fox GM, Joondeph BC, Flynn HW Jr, et al. Delayed-onset pseudophakic endophthalmitis. *Am J Ophthalmol*. 1991;111:163-173.

25. Ficker L, Meredith TA, Wilson LA ,et al. Chronic bacterial endophthalmitis. *Am J Ophthalmol*. 1987;103:745-748.

26. Roussel TJ, Olson ER, Rice T, et al. Chronic postoperative endophthalmitis associated with Actinomyces species. *Arch Ophthalmol*. 1991;109;60-62.

27. Zimmerman PL, Mamalis N, Alder JB, et al. Chronic Nocardia asteroides endophthalmitis after extracapsular cataract extraction. *Arch Ophthalmol*. 1993;111:837-840.

28. Pettit TH, Olson RJ, Foos RY, et al. Fungal endophthalmitis following intraocular lens implantation. *Arch Ophthalmol*. 1980;98:1025-1039.

29. Stern WH, Tamura E, Jacobs RA, et al. Epidemic post-surgical candida parapsilosis endophthalmitis. *Ophthalmology*. 1985;92:1701-1709.

30. Zambrano W, Flynn HW Jr, Pflugfelder SC, et al. Management options for Propionibacterium acnes endophthalmitis. *Ophthalmology*. 1989;96:1100-1105.

31. Winward KE, Pflugfelder SC, Flynn HW Jr, et al. Postoperative propionibacterium endophthalmitis. *Ophthalmology*. 1993;100:447-451.

32. Ciulla TA, Beck AD, Topping TM, et al. Blebitis, early endophthalmitis, and late endophthalmitis after glaucoma-filtering surgery. *Ophthalmology*. 1997;104:986-995.

33. Brown RH, Yang LH, Walker SD, et al. Treatment of bleb infection after glaucoma surgery. *Arch Ophthalmol*. 1994;112:57-61.

34. Mandelbaum S, Forster RK, Gelender H et al. Late onset endophthalmitis associated with filtering blebs. *Ophthalmology*. 1985;92:964-972.

35. Parrish R, Minckler D. Late endophthalmitis-Filtering surgery time bomb? *Ophthalmology*. 1996;103:1167-1168.

36. Wolner B, Liebermann JM, Sassan JW, et al. Late bleb-related endophthalmitis after trabeculectomy with adjunctive 5-fluorouracil. *Ophthalmology*. 1991;98:1053-1060.

37. Higginbotham EJ, Stevens RK, Musch D, et al. Bleb-related endophthalmitis after trabeculectomy with mitomycin C. *Ophthalmology*. 1996;103:650-656.

38. Jett BD, Jensen HG, Atkuri RV, et al. Evaluation of therapeutic measures for treating endophthalmitis caused by isogenic toxin producing and toxin- nonproducing Enterococcus faecalis strains. *Invest Ophthalmol Vis Sci*. 1995;36:9-15.

39. Bohigan GM. Intravitreal antibiotic preparation, pp 64-67. Antifungal agents. pp158-163. In: *External Diseases of the Eye*. Fort Worth, TX: Alcon Laboratories; 1980.

40. Rowsey JJ, Newsom DL, Sexton DJ, et al. Endophthalmitis, current approaches. *Ophthalmology*. 1982;89:1055-1066.

41. Peyman GA, Raichand M, Bennett TO, et al. Management of endophthalmitis with pars plana vitrectomy. *Br J Ophthalmol*. 1980;64:472-475.

This chapter has been reprinted with permission from Chan CC. Postoperative Endophthalmitis. In: Agarwal S, Agarwal A, Agarwal A, ed. *Phacoemulsification*. Jaypee Brothers Medical Publishers (P) Ltd; New Delhi; 2004:482-497.

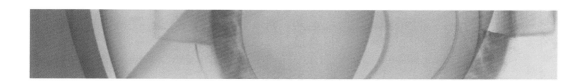

Financial Disclosures

Dr. Amar Agarwal is a consultant for Abbott Medical Optics, Bausch + Lomb, and STAAR Surgical and receives royalties from SLACK Incorporated and Jaypee Highlights.

Dr. Ashvin Agarwal has no financial or proprietary interest in the materials presented herein.

Dr. Athiya Agarwal has no financial or proprietary interest in the materials presented herein.

Dr. Balamurali Krishna Ambati has no financial or proprietary interest in the materials presented herein.

Dr. J. Fernando Arevalo has no financial or proprietary interest in the materials presented herein.

Mr. Fernando A. Arevalo has no financial or proprietary interest in the materials presented herein.

Dr. Clement K. Chan has no financial or proprietary interest in the materials presented herein.

Dr. Garry P. Condon has not disclosed any relevant financial relationships.

Dr. Yassine Daoud has no financial or proprietary interest in the materials presented herein.

Dr. Carlos F. Fernandez has no financial or proprietary interest in the materials presented herein.

Dr. William J. Fishkind is a consultant for Abbott Medical Optics and LensAR and receives royalties from Thieme Publishers.

Dr. Sadeer B. Hannush has no financial or proprietary interest in the materials presented herein.

Dr. Soosan Jacob has no financial or proprietary interest in the materials presented herein.

Dr. Thomas Kohnen has no financial or proprietary interest in the materials presented herein.

Dr. Dhivya Ashok Kumar has no financial or proprietary interest in the materials presented herein.

Dr. Michael Lawless is a member of the Alcon and LenSx USA Medical Advisory Boards.

Dr. Boris Malyugin holds the patent rights for the Malyugin ring.

Dr. Kevin M. Miller has no financial or proprietary interest in the materials presented herein.

Dr. Zoltán Z. Nagy is a consultant to Alcon-LenSx and is a member of the Medical Advisory Board.

Dr. Thomas A. Oetting has no financial or proprietary interest in the materials presented herein.

Dr. Marko Ostovic has no financial or proprietary interest in the materials presented herein.

Dr. Som Prasad is a consultant for Bausch + Lomb and receives travel reimbursement from Alcon.

Dr. Bryce R. Radmall has no financial or proprietary interest in the materials presented herein.

Dr. Shetal M. Raj has no financial or proprietary interest in the materials presented herein.

Dr. Brian C. Stagg has no financial or proprietary interest in the materials presented herein.

Dr. Walter J. Stark has no financial or proprietary interest in the materials presented herein.

Dr. Abhay R. Vasavada has no financial or proprietary interest in the materials presented herein.

Dr. Vaishali A. Vasavada has no financial or proprietary interest in the materials presented herein.

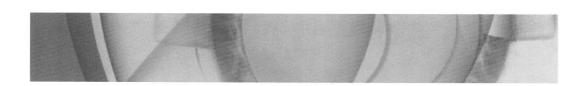

Index

Printed in the United States
by Baker & Taylor Publisher Services